BRENDA BRADSHAW &
LAUREN DONALDSON BRAMLEY, M.D.

the Baby's

OVER 150 EASY, HEALTHY AND TASTY

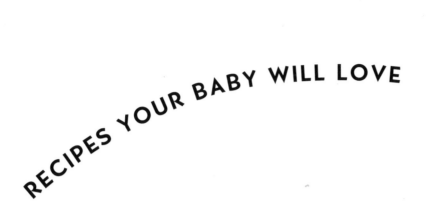

RECIPES YOUR BABY WILL LOVE

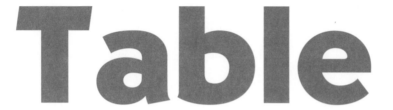

Table

RANDOM HOUSE CANADA

Library and Archives Canada Cataloguing in Publication

Bradshaw, Brenda (Brenda E.)
The baby's table / Brenda Bradshaw & Lauren Donaldson Bramley.—Rev.
and updated.

Includes bibliographical references and index.

ISBN 978–0–307–35883–7

1. Cookery (Baby foods). 2. Infants—Nutrition. I. Bramley,
Lauren Donaldson
II. Title.

RJ216.B663 2010   641.5'6222   C2009–905234–2

Design by CS Richardson

Printed in Canada

2   4   6   8   9   7   5   3   1

To the babies who inspired us,
Charlie, Maxwell, Lachlan,
Owen and Elliotte

Contents

Foreword

As a general consultant pediatrician, I've
been fielding questions for years from new
parents about what (and how) to feed their
children. When I first started my practice, I
am embarrassed to say, many of these questions truly stumped me: When can I stop
warming up the bottle? When can I give the
baby eggs? Juice? Yogurt? It wasn't until I

had children of my own that I realized how much there truly is to learn about the care and feeding of babies. And, alas, knowing how and what to feed a baby and putting it into practice are two different things.

The Baby's Table is full of delicious ideas and recipes. While some of the recipes may sound intimidating to the sleep-deprived new parent (Gourmet Tuna Melts or Salmon and Vegetables with Creamy Dill Sauce), they are all surprisingly simple and quick to prepare. When Mom and Dad are craving their favorite spicy takeout, having some of the dishes frozen in bulk to feed baby is a great option.

This book—part recipe book, part everything-you-need-to-know-to-feed-a-baby—answers all the feeding and nutrition questions I tried to answer in my early years as a pediatrician as well as the questions I had when I was figuring it out for myself as a new parent. The dishes are truly great-tasting as well as nutritious and safe. They focus on unprocessed, unsweetened and unsalted whole foods.

Finally! A book that I will be happy to recommend to new parents, to help them feed their baby for those crucial first years.

Cheryl L. Mutch M.D., C.M., F.R.C.P(C.)
Pediatrician, Burnaby, B.C., Canada

Introduction

If you're like many new parents, you may find the prospect of making your own baby food a daunting one. You're no Naked Chef; baby's keeping you busy (and tired)— and besides, how would you know that what you're feeding your infant is safe and supplies the nutrients needed for healthy development?

It's easier than you think. And *The Baby's Table*, filled with important nutritional information and cooking tips and more than 150 simple and tasty recipes, can show you how. There are helpful hints on dealing with behavioral issues such as feeding problems, and strategies for making healthy eating a pleasurable experience—for you as well as for your baby.

More and more parents today are seeing the advantages of preparing homemade baby food. It's nutritional, economical and takes far less time than you think. All you need is a steamer basket, a blender or food processor, a small double boiler, ice cube trays and a freezer. In an afternoon—during one of baby's naptimes— you can whip up and freeze an entire month's supply of meals rich in essential nutrients.

Your baby's nutrition is of critical importance for physical and intellectual growth and development and has lasting implications for his or her future. Using the tips, recipes and meal plans provided in *The Baby's Table*, you can create your own baby-pleasing fare that offers nutritional advantages not found in commercial brands. Homemade baby food cuts down on unwanted additives and offers your baby a wider variety of textures and flavors than commercial baby food could hope to replicate. The savings are substantial; your own baby food can be prepared at a fraction of the cost of store-bought. In the long term, offering home-prepared baby food can also help you shape your baby's food choices for a healthy childhood, and beyond.

All recipes in *The Baby's Table* have been reviewed by a physician and tested by parents—and more importantly, babies! Information is based on the latest medical and nutritional research and complies with the current Canadian guidelines for infant feeding. Be aware that the contents of this book are not intended as medical advice: the suggestions apply only to healthy, full-term infants, and parents should consult with their doctor before undertaking any change in their infant's diet.

The chapters in *The Baby's Table* are conveniently named for the age group to which the recipes apply: Newborn to Six Months; From Six to Nine Months; From Nine to Twelve Months; and Toddlers. There are also four helpful Appendices: Canada's Food Guide, Resources, Growth Charts, and References. For the purposes of this cookbook, age definitions are as follows: *newborn*, up to one month; *infant*, from birth to 12 months; *toddler*, from 1 to 3 years; and *child*, 3 years and older.

The fact that you're reading this book shows you're ready to take the plunge. Congratulations—you have made a commitment to a healthy future for your baby. Read on, have fun, be creative—and, since you're sure to be taste-testing these recipes yourself, *bon appétit!*

Newborn to Six Months

For the first 6 months your baby will be fed only breast milk or breast milk substitute. The first 6 months is a time of peak growth and bonding, when your baby will double or triple his birth weight, will learn to smile and laugh and will rely on you entirely for healthy nutrition. It has been proven that breast milk is the optimum nutrition for young babies. It is not always possible to breastfeed, however. Regardless of whether it is breast or bottle, a loving and caring approach to feeding will ensure your baby thrives.

BREASTFEEDING

According to the Canadian Paediatric Society, the Dietitians of Canada, Health Canada and the American Academy of Pediatrics, breastfeeding is the optimum method of feeding for all infants with very few exceptions. Research continues to prove the vast benefits of breastfeeding for your baby:

▶ *Reduced rates of infection:* Breastfeeding has been shown to reduce the rates of respiratory, ear, gastrointestinal, urinary tract and other infections in both infancy and childhood by at least 30 to 50 percent. Antibodies and other proteins from the mother prevent infection and strengthen the immune system.

▶ *Possible prevention of Sudden Infant Death Syndrome (SIDS):* In addition to placing an infant on his or her back for sleep, recent studies show a reduced risk of SIDS among breastfed infants.

▶ *Enhanced cognitive development:* Breastfeeding has been shown to improve childhood intelligence quotient (IQ), standardized tests of reading, mathematics and scholastic ability. These improvements are thought in part to be due to the specific fatty acids found only in breast milk.

▶ *Prevention of allergies:* There is evidence to suggest that exclusive breastfeeding for at least the first 3 to 4 months of life is protective against eczema, cow's milk allergy and wheezing in the early years.

▶ *Prevention of iron deficiency:* Breast milk is associated with lower rates of iron deficiency, provided iron-fortified cereals are not postponed much beyond 6 months.

▶ *Other benefits:* There is a possible reduction in asthma, diabetes, bowel diseases and some childhood cancers in breastfed children.

And then there are the health benefits of breastfeeding for mothers:

▶ *Decreased osteoporosis in later life:* During pregnancy, calcium is lost from the mother's bones as a source for the developing baby. The hormones produced by breastfeeding replace the skeletal calcium lost during pregnancy, which leads to a decrease in osteoporosis.

▶ *Decreased cancer risk:* Breastfeeding is associated with a reduced risk of ovarian and breast cancer. This is thought to be due to the reduced levels of estrogen caused by breastfeeding.

▶ *Enhanced weight loss:* Breastfeeding is related to increased weight loss following birth and a faster return to pre-pregnancy weight and body shape. This process begins immediately, as hormones released during breastfeeding promote faster shrinkage of the uterus and mobilization of fat from the lower body. These effects occur without dieting or excessive exercise and are more evident with prolonged breastfeeding.

▶ *Other benefits:* New parents are often overwhelmed by the time commitment of breastfeeding a newborn baby. However, breastfeeding is an excellent way to escape the demands of cleaning, sterilizing and preparing bottles, particularly in the early weeks of baby's life. Furthermore, breast milk is a dynamic substance, which alters its consistency depending on both climate and your baby's needs.

HOW LONG? Many benefits can be achieved with 6 months of exclusive breastfeeding. For this reason Health Canada recommends at least 6 months of exclusive breastfeeding followed by the introduction of nutrient rich complementary foods, with particular attention to iron. It is ideal to continue breastfeeding for the first 2 years and beyond, if possible, as many of the benefits are more marked with prolonged breastfeeding. However, should extended breastfeeding not be possible, the benefits of even a short time are evident.

Eat well and avoid calorie-restricted diets during breastfeeding to ensure adequate energy for milk production. The composition of breast milk will vary according to your diet. The fat-soluble vitamins A, D, E and K and minerals are drawn from storage in your body so that your recent dietary deficiencies are not evident in the breast milk. The water-soluble vitamins C and B-complex are not stored by you and may therefore be deficient in breast milk if you don't meet your dietary needs. Many women choose to continue taking their prenatal vitamin throughout breastfeeding. In some countries, DHA, a type of omega-3 fatty acid, is now included in prenatal vitamins to improve infant brain and eye development and ward off post-natal depression. Speak to your doctor about the possibility of taking a DHA supplement while breastfeeding. If you consume a strict vegetarian diet you will likely be advised by your doctor to take a daily vitamin supplement. All women should drink plenty of fluids while breastfeeding, as it is easy to become dehydrated, which may then lead to exhaustion.

HOW TO GET STARTED Ideally breastfeeding should begin as soon as possible after birth. For the first 48 to 72 hours, breast milk consists only of a clear substance called colostrum. Colostrum is extremely rich in antibodies and plays a crucial role in development of the infant's immune system. As colostrum is low in calories, the breast-fed newborn will lose weight in the first 3 to 4 days of life. Early breastfeeding patterns can be very erratic, and parents may think the baby couldn't possibly be getting enough; however, the infant has a good reserve to help her withstand this early phase. Weight loss is a normal part of early life and it is important for parents not to be discouraged. It is also important to resist supplementing colostrum with formula, or "sugar water" as was once common practice in many hospitals. Today these measures are only taken if medically necessary and are not for normal weight loss alone. The best treatment for the "hungry" baby is more practice at breastfeeding. This also encourages the breast milk to replace colostrum within 2 to 4 days.

In the early weeks newborns should be breastfed whenever they show signs of hunger. Early signs of hunger include increased activity, opening the mouth and turning the head in search of food, or attempting to "latch on." Crying is a late sign of hunger. Once milk has replaced the colostrum, newborns will feed approximately eight to ten times in 24 hours. It is important to hold baby upright for burping following a feed; however, babies may occasionally not burp and need not be continuously patted to do so.

At 1 week of age, adequate breastfeeding is indicated by at least six wet diapers and three to four stools per day. In these early weeks newborns who have not nursed for a period of 4 hours should be roused to feed.

In time, the duration of each feed will become shorter and nursing will occur less frequently. Sometime after the first month, babies may be encouraged to have fewer feeds during night hours with increased duration of morning feeds. This may be accomplished by comforting the baby in other ways, such as holding, rocking or changing.

If discharged from the hospital less than 48 hours after delivery, babies should be evaluated by a health care professional within the first 5 days of life. You should contact your doctor about possible inadequate feeding, the appearance of a yellow tinge to the skin or whites of the eyes (jaundice), vomiting or temperature above 100.4°F/38.0°C.

For concerns regarding breastfeeding, contact your doctor, community nurse or local La Leche League.

VITAMIN SUPPLEMENTATION OF BREASTFED INFANTS Vitamin D is important for normal bone growth and prevention of rickets in children and osteoporosis in adults. It is produced naturally when skin is exposed to sunlight but not always in sufficient quantities. This may be due to decreased exposure to sunlight, use of sunscreen and absence of vitamin D–stimulating rays in northern latitudes during the winter months. To overcome these factors vitamin D has been added to milk, margarine and infant formula in some countries. As breastfed babies do not consume these, they may become deficient in vitamin D.

The Canadian Paediatric Society and the American Academy of Pediatrics have recommended that all breastfed infants in North America be given supplemental vitamin D from birth until they can reliably obtain vitamin D through formula-feeding or vitamin D–fortified milk. Vitamin D supplementation can be given in the form of drops directly to the infant's mouth. This is also recommended for babies in other countries with a northern latitude or limited sunlight, particularly in winter months. According to Health Canada recommendations, all breastfed healthy term infants should receive a Vitamin D supplement of 400 IU daily from birth until the infant's diet includes at least 400 IU from other sources or until the infant reaches 1 year of age. Formula-fed babies may need a vitamin D supplement depending on how much formula they drink. Babies who drink a combination of both breast milk and formula may also need a vitamin D supplement. Research into the importance of vitamin D in cancer prevention, diabetes and obesity is ongoing and recommendations regarding vitamin D supplementation are likely to change. Talk to your doctor regarding an adequate vitamin D dosage.

BISPHENOL A AND BABY BOTTLES

Bisphenol A (BPA) is an industrial chemical used to make polycarbonate, a clear hard plastic that is used in many household products, including baby bottles. It is also found in epoxy resins, which are used to line metal drink and food cans.

Babies tend to have a higher intake of many environmental chemicals, including BPA, because they breathe, drink and eat more on a pound per pound basis than their adult counterparts. They also chew on plastic objects and toys, which may increase their exposure.

Studies indicate that low levels of BPA can affect the development of the nervous system and subsequent behavior in lab animals. There are also indications that BPA may have effects on the prostate gland, mammary glands, and influence earlier onset of puberty for girls. At this point we do not know how these studies relate to human health, and Health Canada states that the levels of BPA in our food and beverage containers are extremely low. Regardless, it makes good sense to limit your family's exposure. This is especially true for infants and young children, whose nervous systems are still developing.

For infants the main exposure comes from pouring hot liquids into polycarbonate baby bottles, as well as from BPA migrating into infant formula from the can's protective lining. Health Canada is moving to ban the sale of polycarbonate bottles. At this point, the best ways to protect your baby is to breastfeed for as long as possible and avoid polycarbonate baby bottles and sippy cups. If using bottles, opt for ones made of glass, stainless steel, or non-BPA plastic. If the bottle is made of hard plastic and has the number 7 in the middle of the recycling symbol, assume it contains BPA. If there is a 7 but no recycling symbol, you cannot be certain it is BPA-free unless you consult the manufacturer. If using glass bottles do not let your baby walk around with them, and be sure to inspect bottles carefully for chips each time you use them. Avoid heating breast milk, formula and food in plastic containers as the heat increases the likelihood that chemicals will leach. Use glass or stainless steel for heating food and always remove formula from the can before heating it. When sterilizing water to make formula, allow water to cool in a non-polycarbonate container prior to pouring it into a plastic bottle. Boiled water can be stored for 2 days in the refrigerator in a tightly closed container. If plastic bottles have been sterilized or washed in the dishwasher, allow them to cool prior to pouring breast milk or formula into them. For more information on BPA, check out Health Canada's website at www.hc-sc.gc.ca.

Many parents wonder about the use of iron supplements for breastfed babies. It is true that iron is present in low quantities in breast milk; however, this iron is easily absorbed by the infant and is adequate for the first 6 months of life. There are also iron stores accumulated in utero. At 6 months iron-fortified cereals should be introduced to offset the depleting iron stores. In pre-term infants and infants with a birth weight less than 5.5 pounds (2.5 kg) it will likely be necessary to provide an iron supplement before 6 months. Again, consult your doctor for a recommended brand and dose.

EXPRESSING AND STORING BREAST MILK Once breastfeeding is well established you can return to work and still provide expressed breast milk for your baby. By using a portable electric, manual or battery-operated breast pump, you can express during breaks and lunch hours. The breast milk can then be stored in sterilized containers in the refrigerator. Many women begin to express and freeze breast milk prior to their anticipated return to work. Breast milk can be stored in the freezer for up to 1 month and in the refrigerator for up to 24 hours. All equipment, storage containers and bottles must be sterilized. For further information contact your doctor, local community nurse or La Leche League.

WARMING THE MILK

Breast milk or formula can be given at body temperature (warm) or cool. Warm the bottle either by running it under warm water or by standing it in a bowl of warm water. Do not heat it on the stovetop as this will cause the bottle to heat up too quickly and can possibly burn your baby's sensitive mouth. Do not use a microwave, as pockets of overheated milk may exist even if the temperature feels fine on your wrist. Furthermore, studies have found that high heat can alter the composition of breast milk and, most importantly, the anti-infective properties of antibodies. There is no need to warm bottles of breast milk or infant formula. On summer days your baby may prefer a chilled bottle.

Studies comparing the cognitive function in babies suggest that those who were breastfed have a developmental advantage and therefore improved cognitive function as measured by IQ tests over those who were formula-fed. This has been attributed in some studies to the long-chain polyunsaturated fatty acids omega-3 and omega-6. Both of these fatty acids are present in breast milk in the form of DHA and AHA. As these fatty acids constitute the majority of the brain and retina it has been proposed that their presence in breast milk is the reason for observed differences in cognitive ability. DHA and AHA have now been synthesized and added to some infant formulas. These formulas have long been available in the U.K., Europe and Australia and more recently in Canada and the U.S. These formulas may have "Omega-3," "DHA" and "AHA" listed in the ingredients.

PRECAUTIONS DURING BREASTFEEDING Certain groups of women may be advised not to breastfeed, including women with active tuberculosis, HIV or AIDS. Review with your doctor the use of any medication, including over-the-counter drugs and herbal remedies.

Nursing women are advised not to exceed minimal and infrequent alcohol consumption while breastfeeding. Alcohol appears in breast milk at similar levels to that in the mother's blood. Small amounts of alcohol render the baby's resultant blood alcohol level very low because of dilution by the baby's body water. Larger quantities, however, may result in harmful blood alcohol levels. Studies have shown impaired motor function of infants whose mothers consume at least one drink each day. Contrary to popular thought, alcohol in breast milk has been shown to decrease infant's sleep and increase wakings within the period following intake. Women who have consumed alcohol are advised to wait at least 1 hour per standard drink prior to breastfeeding to allow some clearance of alcohol from breast milk. Women should not use any illegal drugs such as marijuana, cocaine, heroin and amphetamines at any time while breastfeeding.

FORMULA-FEEDING

Breast milk is the ideal source of nutrition for infants. However, when breastfeeding is not possible, infant formula is the best alternative. For babies who cannot breastfeed and are not being given donor milk, infant formula is the best alternative. Research on improving infant formula continues, particularly in the area of fatty acid supplementation. Only formulas specifically labeled as infant formula should be given to babies less than 1 year of age. There are a number of different brands and preparations of infant formula, but the preparation used by the majority of infants should be iron-fortified formula based on cow's milk. The cow's milk protein used in infants' formula has been isolated and modified from whole cow's milk to a form that is tolerated by infants.

WHAT IS TAURINE?

In an effort to reproduce the benefits of breast milk, taurine has recently been added to some brands of infant formula. This amino acid is found in high levels in the brain, heart and retina, where it performs many important functions. Most notably, taurine is involved in the chemical reactions essential for normal vision, and deficiencies of taurine can cause degradation of the retina. Taurine is found in meat, fish and breast milk and is now often added to infant formula.

IRON-FORTIFIED COW'S MILK PROTEIN-BASED FORMULAS This is the standard breast milk substitute for healthy term infants with no family history of allergies. Brands of formula may differ in whether they contain certain additional compounds equal to those found in breast milk.

SOY PROTEIN-BASED FORMULAS Despite widespread use of soy formulas there are only three indications for its use: a rare metabolic disorder called galactosemia, lactase deficiency, and some vegetarian diets. Furthermore, recent studies suggest that the phytoestrogens (compounds that mimic female hormones) in soy formula may be problematic: they may be linked to adult cancers and may cause younger onset of puberty. The significance of these findings remains unclear and research continues. Using soy protein–based formula unnecessarily may pose certain health risks for your baby. Do not use soy protein–based formula without consulting your doctor.

LACTOSE-FREE COW'S MILK PROTEIN-BASED FORMULAS This formula is used for babies who have been diagnosed as lactose intolerant. Your doctor will confirm this diagnosis through laboratory tests.

PROTEIN HYDROSYLATE FORMULAS (HYPOALLERGENIC FOR-MULAS) These formulas are used only for babies who may be at risk of developing allergies or who have a confirmed allergy to cow's milk proteins or soy proteins. Do not use this formula without a doctor's advice.

FOLLOW-UP FORMULAS Follow-up formulas are designed to be used by infants in the second 6 months of life. Compared with cow's milk, follow-up formulas contain more nutrients and fatty acids and are more readily absorbed. Pasteurized whole cow's milk may be introduced at 12 months of age.

MIXING FORMULA When mixing formula, carefully read and follow the directions on the label.

Ready-to-use formula is sterile until the container is opened. It is ideal for infants who are younger than 1 month, premature or ill. Once opened, the can can be covered and stored in the refrigerator for up to 48 hours. Once the formula is poured into a bottle, it can be stored in the refrigerator for up to 48 hours.

Concentrated liquid formula needs to be mixed with cooled boiled water. Once opened, the can can be covered and stored in the refrigerator for up to 48 hours. Once the formula is prepared, it can be stored in the refrigerator for up to 48 hours.

Powdered infant formula needs to be mixed with cooled boiled water. It is not sterile and in rare cases has made infants ill. If your baby is less than 1 month, premature or ill, do not use powdered formula unless advised to do so by a doctor. Powdered formula needs to be stored in a cool, dry place, not in the refrigerator. Check the expiry date and use the formula within a month of opening it. Keep formula prepared from powder in the refrigerator for no longer than 24 hours.

When taking breast milk or formula on the go use an ice pack and insulated container to keep it cool. Discard any unused milk that has been left out at room temperature for more than 2 hours. If milk has been heated or partially drunk, throw it out after an hour. Do not put it in the refrigerator to re-use.

BOTTLE STERILIZATION Correct preparation, cleaning and sterilization of all bottles and storage containers for expressed breast milk and formula are critical for the safety of your baby. Bacteria can grow in breast milk or formula and may cause gastroenteritis. All equipment must be thoroughly cleaned and then sterilized either on the stovetop or with a microwave or electric sterilization unit. Sterilization should continue until at least 4 months of age for a healthy, full-term baby. At this time your baby's gastrointestinal system should be able to kill the bacteria.

BABY BOTTLE NIPPLES Baby bottle nipples should be inspected before and after each use because tears and holes may appear with age and as a result of heat exposure. Discard nipples once they show signs of wear and tear to prevent your baby from choking on broken nipple pieces.

WATER Water used to prepare infant formula or baby food, and water offered for drinking must be free of chemical and microbiological contamination. Water used for mixing infant formula must be boiled in a clean open pot for 2 minutes and then cooled with the lid on. This applies to bottled water, home filtered water and well water. Make sure you allow the water to cool if pouring it into a plastic bottle as the heat may cause chemicals from the plastic to leach into the water. If you have concerns about your water or are on a well system, check with your local public health unit about the safety of your water supply.

▶ *Tap Water:* When using tap water, allow the tap to run freely for 2 minutes each morning to flush out contaminants such as lead and copper that may have accumulated overnight. Also, use only water from the cold water tap as hot water may leach more contaminants from pipes.

▶ *Commercially Bottled Non-Carbonated Water:* Commercially bottled waters suitable for use by infants are natural spring water drawn from underground springs and treated water, both of which have low mineral content. Mineral water, treated water with a high mineral content, and carbonated water are not suitable as they may be difficult for the infant's kidneys to metabolize.

▶ *Home Water Filters:* Home water treatment can be used to filter tap water but may pose additional problems. Charcoal filters may be a source of bacterial or silver contamination, and some softeners may add excess sodium. To enquire about your home water treatment equipment, contact the Criteria Section, Bureau of Chemical Standards, Health Canada (see Appendix II, page 191).

FLUORIDE

Fluoridation of the water supply is the most effective way to prevent dental cavities. However, many parts of Canada and other countries do not have fluoridated water. Recommended levels of fluoride have trended downwards in the past 10 years in an effort to reduce the incidence of dental fluorosis. Dental fluorosis occurs as a result of excessive fluoride exposure. It is characterized by white streaks or specks or brown-gray staining of the teeth. The teeth remain resistant to cavities and there are no health consequences of fluorosis. Recently there has been an increase in dental fluorosis from increased exposure to fluoride through the additive effects of fluoridated water, fluoride supplements, foods and drinks made with fluoridated water, toothpaste and mouthwashes. Fluorosis is now seen in up to 60 percent of children.

Age of Child	Fluoride Concentration of Principal Drinking Water	
	◄ 0.3 ppm	► 0.3 ppm
0 to 6 mths	None	None
6 mths to 3 yrs	0.25 mg/day	None
3 to 6 yrs	0.5 mg/day	None
6 yrs	1 mg/day	None

RECOMMENDED SUPPLEMENTAL FLUORIDE CONCENTRATIONS FOR CHILDREN

Source: Canadian Paediatric Society: *Paediatrics & Child Health 2002;* 7(8):569–572, Reference no. N02-01. Revision in progress 2009.

To determine the fluoride content of your water supply, contact your doctor, dentist or local water authority office.

OTHER FLUIDS Fruit juice is an excellent source of vitamin C, but should not be introduced until the second year to avoid it becoming a substitute for breast milk or infant formula. Furthermore, excessive juice intake may be a cause of failure to thrive or chronic diarrhea. If offering juice, do not dilute it with water. The recommended daily allowance of vitamin C for infants aged 6 to 12 months is 20 mg and is easily provided in breast milk, formula, fruits and vegetables. Babies less than 1 year may be offered water once they are well established on breast milk or formula and gaining weight well. They do not require extra water in addition to breast milk or formula except in hot weather.

COLIC Colic is defined as excessive crying in healthy infants that persists for at least 3 hours, on at least 3 days per week, for at least 3 weeks. Colic is thought to occur in approximately 13 percent of infants and usually begins at 3 to 4 weeks of age and persists until the infant is about 3 to 4 months of age. Although there are many theories, the cause of colic remains unknown, as does the cure.

When faced with excessive crying it is important to ask the following questions: Is baby hungry, cold, hot or in pain? Provided your baby is healthy, thriving and not found to have any abnormality on examination by your doctor, it is possible he may have colic. During crying spells both parents and baby endure significant stress. There are no medications or remedies that have been proven safe and effective to relieve crying. Parents are encouraged to try stroking, massaging, rocking and cuddling the infant. There is no evidence to support changing to soy formula to relieve colic; however, your doctor may suggest a week-long trial of a protein hydrosylate formula if baby is formula-fed.

As crying spells can be extremely upsetting to parents, it is important to request assistance from friends and relatives in caring for a baby with colic. If you ever feel "at the end of your rope," contact your doctor immediately.

WEANING is the introduction of foods other than breast milk. This may be whole cow's milk (if over 12 months) or formula (if exclusive breastfeeding is no longer possible). Milk or formula will now be delivered by cup or bottle and will taste very different from breast milk. It is best to make the transition slowly to allow a smooth adjustment for both baby and parent. Weaning may begin by replacing the baby's least favorite feed per day with formula or whole cow's milk. For each subsequent week, replace an additional daily feed. This process may take 4 to 6 weeks or longer, depending on your baby.

BREAST MILK AND IMMUNIZATIONS

At the ages of 2, 4, 6, 12 and 18 months, your doctor will offer your baby immunizations. It has been recognized that breastfed babies may develop a stronger immunity to some diseases and are presumably better protected. This response is just one of the many benefits of breastfeeding and is thought to be because of the fatty acids present in breast milk. One of these fatty acids, linoleic acid, has recently been added to some infant formulas and improved immunity has also been seen in babies fed these formulas.

From Six to Nine Months

Your baby is showing an increased interest in the food you are eating and seems unsatisfied after feeds. You've also noticed that she's able to hold her head up and sit in an upright position.

The time has come: she's ready for solid food. Your *homemade* food.

PREPARING BABY FOOD

Making baby food is easy. To get started, all you need is the following:
- this book
- steamer basket (or multi-layer steamer)
- blender or food processor (a handheld immersion blender can also be useful)
- ice cube trays
- freezer bags and labels
- freezer
- double-boiler
- tinfoil or parchment paper
- and, of course, a hungry baby!

Steaming is the method of choice for cooking fruits and vegetables as it preserves their fresh taste, vitamin content and even color. You'll need a blender or food processor to purée the food to suit your baby's age and desired texture. You will find a handheld immersion blender convenient for puréeing smaller quantities of food. Once puréed, simply pour the food into ice cube trays, cover with tinfoil or parchment paper, freeze, and later transfer the food cubes to labeled freezer bags. When your baby is hungry, preparing a meal is as easy as defrosting a cube.

Before you get started, here are a few things to keep in mind:

▶ *Hygiene:* Cleanliness is extremely important when preparing food for your family. Prior to making baby food, wash your hands thoroughly with soap and warm water, and ensure that the equipment and the cooking areas are clean. Equipment and utensils should be thoroughly hand washed using hot water and detergent, or cleaned in a dishwasher on a high heat setting. All fruits and vegetables, including those being peeled, should be thoroughly washed. This is because surface bacteria on the skin comes into contact with the knife or peeler.

▶ *Get fresh:* When making food for your baby, always use the freshest ingredients.

▶ *Do it right:* Always ensure that food is correctly cooked before freezing it or serving it to your baby.

▶ *Straining or puréeing:* Because of concerns about baby's choking, many experts advocate straining food for your infant's first few months. If your baby seems to be struggling with new textures, use a sieve: place 1/2 cup of cooked food in the sieve and press with the back of a spoon.

▶ *Freezing and storage:* After preparing any of the bulk recipes in *The Baby's Table*, pour the food into ice cube trays, cover with tinfoil or parchment paper and freeze. If using plastic ice cube trays, allow the food to cool before pouring it into the ice cube trays. This is because heat increases the likelihood that chemicals from the plastic will leach into your baby's food. Alternatively, you can use stainless steel ice cube trays. Once cubes of food are frozen, they can be stored in airtight freezer bags. These should be carefully labeled and dated. Frozen baby food can be stored for up to 2 months in the freezer, and, once thawed, will keep for 48 hours in the refrigerator.

▶ *Thawing:* Baby food should always be thawed in the refrigerator, or in a double boiler on the stovetop, never by leaving it out on the counter at room temperature. Proper thawing prevents the possibility of bacteria growing on the outer layer while the inner core is still frozen. Baby food does not need to be heated prior to serving. On summer days your baby may enjoy a chilled purée. If you choose to warm your baby's food, remember it should be no warmer than body temperature (37°C/98.6°F). This is because babies are used to the temperature of breast milk. Food can be warmed in either the double boiler that was used for defrosting or in a saucepan over low heat. Before serving, remember to mix thoroughly and test in order to avoid hot spots. The most effective way to gauge the temperature of baby food is to test it yourself. Once food has been served, leftovers should be discarded because bacteria from the mouth will have contaminated the food. A microwave is not advised for warming as dangerous hot spots are much more likely to occur than with other methods of heating.

▶ *Cooking times and quantities:* For the recipes in this book, quantities are approximate and most are measured using a standard-size ice cube tray. The number of cubes your baby will eat in a month varies depending on age, individual appetite and how often you choose to supplement the cubes. Supplemental foods include whole-grain infant cereals, finger foods and table foods as your baby grows. When your baby is 6 months old you might make only two recipes: one beef and one vegetable. You will need two ice cube trays and it will take approximately 20 minutes. By the time your baby is 10 months old you may be making four to six recipes per month: one meat, one pasta, one fish and two vegetables. Depending on the complexity of the recipes and how many you make, it will take approximately 1 to 3 hours and you will probably need six to eight ice cube trays. If you have a very hungry baby, be prepared to invest in additional ice cube trays. As your baby gets older, muffin tins work just as well, producing larger portions. Cooking times too will vary.

▶ *Allergy alert:* The recipes in the following chapters adhere to accepted guidelines for introducing foods to your baby. For more information on allergies, see the sections Starting Solids, and Adverse Reactions and Allergies, next.

STARTING SOLIDS

The recommended age to start your baby on solid foods has changed dramatically over the years and in various countries. Recommendations for the introduction of particular food groups

SIGNS YOUR BABY MAY BE READY TO START SOLID FOODS

- Baby is consistently waking more frequently in the night.
- Baby is interested in the foods you are eating.
- Baby seems unsatisfied after feeds.
- Baby frequently seems bored or disinterested in feeds.
- Baby is crying more often between feeds.
- Baby is falling off growth curves on plots of weight measurements.
- Baby is able to sit in an upright position and to hold his head up.

have also varied considerably. Our recommendations in *The Baby's Table* are based on *Nutrition for Healthy Term Infants*, the statement of the Joint Working Group of the Canadian Paediatric Society, the Dietitians of Canada and Health Canada. These recommendations are based on two things: maximizing the time the infant spends exclusively breastfeeding, and ensuring the infant is physiologically mature enough to digest solid foods.

The age of 6 months is the ideal time to introduce solid foods. Introducing food then is thought to minimize the risk of gastro-intestinal infections. On the other hand, if parents wait until their infants are much older than 6 months, the baby runs the risk of developing iron-deficiency anemia as his fetal stores gradually become depleted. Furthermore, a number of studies have shown that there is no real nutritional advantage in introducing solids at an earlier age.

Your baby, like every baby, is unique and will be ready to begin eating solids at a different time from your best friend's baby or the baby next door. Watch for the signs mentioned in the sidebar above. If your baby demonstrates these signs, it may be reasonable to begin solids a little earlier. Consult your doctor or health care professional if you suspect your baby is hungry and might benefit from beginning solids before 6 months. If this is the case, be sure to breastfeed before giving any solids so he will continue to get lots of your milk while his diet is transitioning.

25

On the other hand some healthy, full-term infants are not quite neurologically ready for the complex tongue movements needed to eat solids. They will indicate this by pushing food out of their mouths—the tongue extrusion reflex. If this is the case, continue to offer solids at your baby's pace. Let your baby taste and play with the food. This is an important learning experience. Be reassured that soon he will be gobbling up all kinds of food. Babies born prematurely often have to wait until they reach the age of 6 months past their normal due date before starting solids. Whatever the case, continue to have your baby weighed regularly so that your health care professional can monitor his growth to ensure a healthy transition to solid foods. If your baby is not well onto solids by 9 months, see your doctor, as it may be necessary to test for iron-deficiency anemia.

Start solids when your baby is interested, content and alert. Begin by serving solids two to three times per day and increase to three to four feedings per day. Initial feedings are for practice and pleasure only. If your baby resists these first attempts, do not be disappointed. Try again another day. Breast milk or formula still constitute the majority of calories and nutrients, anyway, so only offer small amounts of solid food at a relaxed pace. Start with 1 tablespoon, mixed with breast milk or formula, and slowly increase the quantity as your baby desires. Observe your baby's cues of satiety and hunger. Do not overfeed or persist if baby seems full or uninterested.

Current recommendations state that high iron foods such as single-grain, iron-fortified infant cereal or well-cooked, finely minced meat, poultry and fish be introduced first. To make meats more palatable, mix them with breast milk, formula and/or leftover cooking water. When introducing a new food, serve it either on its own or with a familiar favorite, as this is the best way to monitor for allergies and/or adverse reactions.

Typically, iron-fortified single-grain infant cereals are the first food introduced and there are no homemade substitutes. These cereals are unlikely to cause allergies, are easily digested and have been fortified to replenish iron stores. A good first choice is iron-fortified rice cereal followed at weekly intervals by barley, oatmeal and, finally, wheat. It is best to introduce wheat last as wheat is associated with an increased incidence of allergies. After you have introduced all the grains individually, you can start introducing mixed cereals. Iron-fortified infant cereals will form the basis of your baby's diet for the first 2 years of life, and will help to ensure adequate iron intake.

Once your baby has mastered infant cereals and meats, it is time to introduce vegetables and fruits. Because infant cereals and meats are rich in iron, it is important to continue serving them while introducing the new foods. Once your baby is eating a variety of vegetables and fruits you can begin mixing them together and with meats to make a number of delicious combinations. This is also the time to introduce lentils, legumes and eggs, as these foods are also considered good sources of iron.

From 6 to 9 months your infant is learning how to bite, chew and swallow. During this period most babies transition from eating food that is puréed smooth and quite runny in consistency to more textured purées, finger foods and even table foods eaten by the rest of the family. Some babies will make this transition in a couple of months; for others it takes longer. How quickly your baby moves through these stages is simply developmental. You can encourage your baby by gradually introducing a variety of new foods with different textures.

At around 9 months your baby should be exposed to a wide variety of different foods. At this stage, the recipes become more complex and involve combinations of several food groups. This is a reasonable time to introduce dairy products, including cottage cheese, plain yogurt and shredded pieces of hard cheese, like cheddar or Gouda and pasteurized soft cheeses. Whole cow's milk for drinking should be postponed until 12 months of age. Introducing dairy products much earlier is associated with an increased risk of gastrointestinal bleeding.

It is not advised to add infant cereal or puréed food to your baby's bottle, which may increase the risk of choking and aspiration. There is no convincing evidence to suggest that adding cereal at bedtime will help your baby sleep through the night.

The recipes in this book are laid out in a suggested order of introduction. The recommendations apply to healthy, full-term infants who do not have a family history of atopic disease (allergies, asthma and eczema). Certain foods must always be avoided in infancy (see the chart entitled Proceed with Caution on page 62).

ADVERSE REACTIONS AND ALLERGIES

Adverse reactions to food commonly occur in the first year of life and many will resolve on their own by 3 years of age. Up to one-third of all children will have an adverse reaction to food characterized by any of the following symptoms: vomiting, diarrhea, skin rashes, itching, runny nose, congestion or wheezing. Although allergies are on the rise, most adverse reactions to food are food intolerances rather than true allergies. Adverse reactions may also occur as a reaction to a chemical in the food.

The specific term "food intolerance" refers to a sensitivity to a specific food, not involving the immune system. Food intolerances originate in the gastrointestinal tract and are often caused by the inability to absorb or digest certain foods. The most common food intolerances are lactose intolerance and celiac disease.

Lactose intolerance occurs when there is insufficient lactase, the enzyme needed to digest the naturally occurring sugar (lactose) found in all types of milk, including breast milk. Congenital lactose intolerance is rare in infancy, but lactase activity declines dramatically throughout childhood, and some children will develop an intolerance. Symptoms include bloating, diarrhea and abdominal pain. If you suspect your baby is lactose intolerant, see your doctor. Lactose intolerance is most common among those of Asian, African American and First Nations descent. It can also develop temporarily after an episode of gastroenteritis, commonly known as the stomach flu.

Celiac disease is an inherited intolerance to gluten, the protein found in wheat, rye and barley. (Some people with celiac disease are also sensitive to oats.) Symptoms of celiac disease may include pain, gas, bloating, indigestion, recurrent diarrhea and constipation. Some infants and children will have poor growth and development, irritability or unexplained anemia. If celiac disease runs in your family, you may want to watch your infant closely and talk with your doctor if symptoms develop after adding wheat to your baby's diet.

A chemical sensitivity occurs when a person has an adverse reaction to a chemical found in a particular food. People with chemical sensitivities may react to caffeine, artificial food dyes, sodium benzoate and/or monosodium glutamate to name just a few. One of the easiest ways to avoid chemical sensitivities is to serve your baby whole foods and avoid highly processed foods as much as possible.

Unlike a food intolerance or chemical sensitivity, food allergies or "food hypersensitivity" involve the immune system. True food allergies affect an estimated 6 percent of children, many of whom will outgrow their allergies—it is estimated that only 3 to 4 percent of adults have food allergies. A food allergy occurs when the immune system mistakenly tries to defend itself against a food protein. Allergic reactions range from mild to severe and symptoms may include itchy eyes, skin rashes, cramps, diarrhea, vomiting, wheezing and shortness of breath, tongue and facial swelling, drop in blood pressure, rapid heartbeat and even loss of consciousness.

Although any food can cause an allergy, the vast majority of allergies are caused by ten foods: peanuts, tree nuts (including almonds, Brazil nuts, hazelnuts, cashews, pecans, pine nuts, macadamia nuts, walnuts and pistachios), sesame seeds, milk, eggs, fish, shellfish, soy,

THE HYGIENE HYPOTHESIS

The hygiene theory is one possible explanation for the sudden rise in allergies. This theory suggests that if a child is kept too clean he has a greater risk of developing allergies. The idea being that, if a child is exposed to certain viral and bacterial illnesses early in life, his immune system will be stimulated to fight the diseases rather than develop allergies. It seems that children who go to daycare from an early age, have more than three siblings, are exposed to animals and come from a lower socioeconomic background seem to have lower rates of allergies. There is still much to be learned about the hygiene hypothesis, but it is certainly food for thought.

wheat and sulphites. Fortunately it is rare for children to have serious allergies to more than two or three foods. Diagnosis of an allergy requires a careful analysis of the diet and symptoms and, if necessary, specific tests to confirm the allergy. If a food allergy is diagnosed your doctor will recommend removing the offending food from the diet. When your child is older, and it is suspected that your child has outgrown his allergy, an allergist may consider performing a food challenge. A food challenge must never be attempted without medical supervision.

In most cases the development of an allergy depends on a genetic predisposition. Your infant is considered high risk for food allergies if he has a parent, brother or sister with atopic disease (eczema, allergies or asthma). It is possible for a parent to have hay fever and their children to develop food allergies. Until recently, parents had been advised to delay the introduction of certain foods in hopes of preventing allergies. This advice was based on expert opinion and not on scientific evidence. There is no convincing evidence to suggest that delaying the foods beyond 6 months will prevent allergies. Today, cases are looked at on an individual basis. If your baby has shown no signs of any adverse reactions to food, does not have eczema or asthma and is not considered at risk for developing allergies, there is no reason to further delay the introduction of these foods beyond 6 months. However, if your infant has experienced any adverse reaction to food (including breast milk or formula), has eczema and/or you have a family history of atopic disease (eczema, allergies and asthma), see your doctor or health care professional to discuss the introduction of solid foods. They may recommend you delay the introduction of certain foods until your baby is better able to communicate any distress she may be feeling.

Regardless of when you decide to introduce specific foods, you should be aware of the ten foods which typically cause allergies. When introducing these foods serve them on their own in small amounts as this is the best way to monitor your baby's reaction. Introduce them in the morning or at lunch so that if your baby does react it doesn't happen in the middle of the night. Some symptoms occur immediately after eating the offending food, while others can take several hours to days to appear. And whatever you do, don't offer these foods when camping or in an isolated location away from access to medical care.

PEANUTS Peanut allergy occurs in an estimated 1 percent of children, and most children who have it do not outgrow it. Peanuts can cause a serious reaction called anaphylaxis. Anaphylaxis causes swelling of the mouth and throat and/or collapse and shock. Anaphylaxis is a life-threatening emergency: seek medical attention immediately. For children diagnosed with peanut allergy, strict avoidance of all peanut products is mandatory.

Any child diagnosed with a severe food allergy should have a Medic Alert bracelet identifying the allergy and should always have caregivers who are informed and prepared to manage an anaphylactic reaction. Doctors usually recommend that children keep with them a dose of epinephrine in an easy-to-use "pen" injector. Should anaphylaxis occur, the medication should be administered immediately. Fatalities have occurred when children were inadvertently given the food and medication was not administered immediately. Because of the severity of peanut allergy, you may choose to wait a little longer before introducing peanut products. This way, your baby will be better able to communicate any discomfort.

TREE NUTS Tree nuts are not related to peanuts, and it is possible to be allergic to peanuts without being allergic to tree nuts. However, many children who are allergic to peanuts are also allergic to tree nuts. For these children strict avoidance of all nuts is often recommended. Most tree nuts are processed in plants where peanuts are also processed, so for safety's sake, you must assume that all tree nuts are contaminated with peanuts.

EGGS Egg allergy is generally caused by the protein found in egg whites. Most children diagnosed with egg allergy will outgrow it by their fifth birthday.

Because eggs are common ingredients in many foods, careful analysis of ingredient lists is needed to avoid eggs. Avoiding eggs means avoiding "egg substitutes" and any foods that list albumin, globulin, ovomucin or vitellin. Egg products were once used in the production of the MMR (measles, mumps and rubella) vaccine, although newer versions of the vaccine are egg-product free. Flu shots also may contain egg products. Although allergic reactions to vaccines are very rare, always advise your doctor prior to vaccination if there is an egg allergy or family history of food allergies.

COW'S MILK Cow's milk allergy is one of the most common food allergies among infants. However most will outgrow it by the age of 3 or 4. It is generally caused by one or more of the proteins found in milk. Symptoms may include stomach cramps, difficulty breathing, rashes, vomiting and diarrhea. If breastfeeding, you may need to eliminate dairy products from your diet because the offending protein can pass into your breast milk. If formula-feeding, whey-protein hydrosylate formula is a better alternative to cow's milk protein–based formula for infants at risk for milk allergy. Soy formula should not be used as it is also possible to develop an allergy to soy. If you suspect your baby has or is at risk for a cow's milk allergy, see your doctor.

WHEAT Wheat is the most common grain allergy. Because of this, it has traditionally been recommended that the introduction of wheat be delayed until other grain cereals have been introduced. Wheat is a "hidden" ingredient in many foods such as processed cheese, soy sauce and battered fish sticks. Careful analysis of ingredients is required to avoid it.

SESAME SEEDS Sesame seed allergies can be severe, even causing anaphylaxis.

SHELLFISH AND FISH Fish allergies can be severe and most children do not outgrow them.

SOY Soy allergy is fairly common in infancy, however many children will eventually outgrow it. Avoiding soy can be difficult as it is a common ingredient in many commercial products, including processed meats, baked goods, breakfast cereals, margarine, drinks and ice cream. To avoid soy, carefully read all ingredient lists.

SULPHITES Sulphites are used as a preservative and can be found in a wide variety of foods, including dried, frozen and canned fruits and vegetables, as well as processed meat, condiments and baked goods. If you suspect your baby is sensitive to sulphites, read labels carefully and consult your doctor.

If you are advised to avoid giving your baby certain foods, you need to be aware of all foods that may contain the offending ingredient.

Full lists of all hidden sources, food labeling and safe alternatives can be obtained from the American Academy of Allergy, Asthma and Immunology (see Appendix II, page 191).

BABY'S FIRST FOODS

It wasn't long ago that we recommended introducing fruit and vegetables before meat. But because iron-deficiency anemia is a common finding among infants between the ages of 6 and 24 months, foods containing iron, such as well-cooked meat, poultry and fish, are now introduced before vegetables and fruit.

What follows are simple meat, chicken and fish recipes that are ideal for your baby's first meals. These recipes will need to be puréed smooth and served almost runny in consistency. This can be achieved by adding leftover cooking water and/or breast milk or formula. When adding liquids, start slowly and add just enough to thin out the purée. If baby rejects it the first time, you may want to add a little more liquid or even mix it with rice cereal to make it more palatable.

After introducing meats you can add other iron-containing foods such as legumes, egg yolks and tofu, as well as fruit and vegetables to your baby's diet. It is important, however, to keep serving iron-fortified infant cereals and meat, since iron from meat sources is more readily absorbed than iron from plant sources. Once a variety of fruit and vegetables is added to your baby's diet you can begin mixing them with meat to make the assortment of delicious recipes found in this book.

First Meats and Fish

In addition to being a good source of iron, meats and fish also contain protein and fat. Fat is an essential component of your baby's diet. It provides a dense source of calories for energy, insulates against the cold, facilitates the absorption of fat-soluble vitamins (A, D, E and K) and constitutes a major part of the developing nervous system. Protein, for its part, provides the building blocks necessary to build and repair body tissues.

POACHED CHICKEN BREAST

Poaching is the ideal way to cook chicken for your baby. This method tenderizes the meat while it cooks and also eliminates the possibility of charring that can occur with grilling or broiling. Charred food contains known carcinogens and should be avoided. Use this recipe as the basis for the puréed chicken recipes that follow.

I chicken breast
I sprig fresh tarragon (optional)

• In shallow frying pan, place chicken breast flat and add water to cover and tarragon (if using). Bring water to a boil, then cover pan with tinfoil and reduce heat to a simmer for 5 minutes. Flip breast and continue to simmer for another 5 to 7 minutes, depending on the size of the breast. Allow chicken to cool in water. The meat should be firm to touch and white throughout. There should be no trace of pink and the juices should run clear.

BABY'S FIRST CHICKEN PURÉE

If you aren't using formula and don't have extra breast milk, you can use extra poaching water to further thin out this purée.

I recipe Poached Chicken Breast
  (page 36)
I/2 cup leftover poaching water
I/4 cup breast milk or formula,
  (approx)

• Place chicken in food processor and purée slowly adding water. Continue to purée adding milk as needed until smooth. Add extra milk if needed.

Yield: 8 cubes

BABY'S FIRST BEEF PURÉE

The method of choice for cooking red meat is stewing, as it tenderizes the meat while it cooks. Ideally, opt for boneless chuck because it is marbled with fat. Fat not only tenderizes the meat, but is essential for your baby's developing brain. This recipe can be made with either beef or lamb. If you aren't using formula and don't have extra breast milk, you can use extra cooking water to further thin out this purée.

I lb stewing beef

I 1/2 cups water

1/4 cup breast milk or formula
   (approx)

• Place meat and water in a saucepan and bring to a boil. Reduce heat and simmer until beef is cooked through, about 20 minutes.

• With a slotted spoon, remove beef and place in food processor. Set aside leftover cooking water.
• Purée slowly adding 1/2 cup leftover cooking water. Continue to purée, adding milk as needed until smooth. Add extra milk if needed.

Yield: 14 to 16 cubes

DID YOU KNOW?

Before a baby is born she is exposed to many flavors. This is because the foods the mother eats during pregnancy can affect the smell of the amniotic fluid. Furthermore, a recent study suggests that childhood taste preferences are shaped by the sweetness of breast milk or formula in the first few months. Most interestingly in breastfed babies, childhood taste preferences also seem to be influenced by the foods the mother ate while she was breastfeeding.

BABY'S FIRST FISH PURÉE

Fish is a potential allergen so if your baby has shown any adverse reaction to food (including breast milk or formula) or is considered at high risk for developing allergies, you should talk to your doctor before introducing it.

Baking in tinfoil is the simplest way to cook fish—allowing it to cook in its own juices. The easiest way to remove the skin is to cook the fish with the skin intact and then gently remove it when done. When done, fish will be firm to touch, opaque throughout and flake easily with a fork.

When serving fish to a baby you must check carefully for bones. The only way to be sure there are no bones is to flake the cooked fish apart with your fingers. You can never be too careful about bones when serving fish to your baby.

10 oz sole fillet

1/3 cup breast milk or formula
   (approx)

• Place fish on tinfoil. Wrap and bake in 375°F oven until thoroughly cooked, about 20 minutes.
• Open foil and allow to cool. Flake fish apart with fingers to remove skin and bones.

• Place fish and cooking juices in food processor and purée. Slowly add milk if needed and purée until smooth. If mixture seems too thick add extra milk to achieve desired consistency.

Yield: 8 cubes

Vegetables and Fruit

Vegetables and fruit are rich in the carbohydrates, vitamins, minerals and disease-fighting antioxidants your growing baby needs. Vegetables should also be valued for their high mineral content, most notably calcium, iron and zinc. Because many babies have an innate preference for sweeter tasting foods, it makes sense to establish a love for vegetables before introducing fruit. The root vegetables are naturally sweet and therefore a good place to start. Mixing root vegetables with the stronger tasting green vegetables will increase their palatability.

From single-fruit mash to mixed fruit smoothies, fruit will likely be a hit with your baby. The high level of vitamin C in fruit promotes healthy growth of skin and bones, and facilitates iron absorption from other foods. Best of all, the natural sugars appeal to babies' developing taste buds.

It is important to choose well-ripened fruit, which is sweeter in flavor and easier on the digestive system than less ripe fruit. Fruit can be served steamed and puréed, simply puréed or even mashed. Softer fruit such as bananas, avocados, papayas, peaches and melons are obvious choices for mashing. Mixing any combination of fresh fruit with a little unsweetened apple juice makes a delicious fruit salad. Oranges and other citrus fruit are acidic, however, and should not be introduced until after 12 months. Though fresh fruit is best, you can choose to introduce canned fruit or frozen fruit. If buying canned, make sure it has been packed in juice with no added sugar.

Dried fruit is rich in iron and has a high fiber content, and therefore functions as a natural laxative. Baby's dried fruit should be stewed for 25 minutes and then puréed. As dried fruit has a concentrated sugar content, it is important to clean baby's teeth afterward. This can be done with either a damp washcloth or a baby toothbrush, depending on the infant's age.

Steaming is the method of choice for cooking both vegetables and fruit because it preserves their great taste and vitamin content. As your baby moves through the 6 to 9 month period you can cut down on the cooking time to preserve nutrient content. Initially your baby will require runny purées. This can be achieved by adding leftover cooking water, breast milk or formula, unsweetened apple juice, homemade vegetable stock (recipe, page 58) or even tap water to the purée. When doing so, add 1 tablespoon at a time to achieve desired consistency. During this period your baby will move from purées to more textured foods. As your baby makes this transition, use the food processor in short pulses to aid with mixing and chopping. A fork can also be used to mash cooked vegetables and soft fruits. The majority of the following purées can be made in bulk and frozen.

GROWTH DIFFERENCES

Breastfed babies tend to be slightly leaner than formula-fed infants; however, they catch up once solids are established. The difference in growth rates is likely because of the difference in fat and protein contents of breast milk and formula. Breast milk adapts to baby's age and to climate, to provide adequate nutrition depending on growth and caloric needs. This difference is entirely normal and expected provided your baby is growing and thriving. Plot your baby's height and weight on a standardized growth curve to follow his development through the first year (see Appendix III, page 195).

LUSCIOUS YAMS

This purée can also be made with sweet potatoes.

4 yams, washed, peeled and
  blemishes removed
1/2 cup of leftover cooking water
  (approx)

• Cut the yams into cubes.
• In steamer, cook yams over boiling water until tender, about 20 to 30 minutes. Set leftover cooking water aside.
• In blender or food processor, purée yams, adding leftover cooking water as needed to achieve desired consistency.
• Pour into ice cube trays and freeze.

Yield: 19 to 20 cubes

BENEFITS OF BETA-CAROTENE

Beta-carotene is a phytochemical that acts as an antioxidant and thereby reduces the risk of some cancers in adults. It is found in yellow, orange and red fruit and vegetables. Studies have indicated it may help to reduce heart disease and improve arthritis in adults—and research is continuing. Although supplements are available, their long-term safety has not been adequately studied. For now, the best sources of beta-carotene are carrots, pumpkin, squash, sweet potatoes, cantaloupe, mango and papaya. It is possible for babies to eat an excess of beta-carotene and develop a harmless condition called hyper-carotenemia, characterized by an orange pigmentation of the skin and hair. Remember, it is better to provide your baby with a wide variety of fruit and vegetables.

CARROTS

Baby carrots are best as they are sweeter and are more likely to appeal.

8 baby carrots, washed, peeled
    and sliced

• In steamer, steam carrots over boiling water for 15 minutes. Set leftover cooking water aside.
• In blender or food processor, purée until smooth, adding leftover cooking water as needed.
• Pour into ice cube trays and freeze.

Yield: 8 to 10 cubes

BUTTERNUT SQUASH

Butternut squash is naturally sweet and another vegetable that will probably make your baby's top ten favorite foods list.

I butternut squash, washed

• Peel skin using a sharp paring knife. Cut squash in half, remove seeds and section.
• In steamer, cook over boiling water until tender, 10 to 12 minutes. Set leftover cooking water aside.
• In blender or food processor, purée squash until smooth, adding leftover cooking water if needed.
• Pour into ice cube trays and freeze.

Yield: 10 cubes

BANANA

Typically, banana is the first raw fruit you will feed your baby. Once the infant is ready to move on, banana blends well with other fruit (because of its creamy texture) to make delicious fruit combinations. Try mixing mashed banana with a cube of your baby's favorite fruit purée.

GREEN BEANS

2 handfuls green beans, washed,
   ends and stringy bits removed

• In steamer, cook beans over boiling water for 10 to 12 minutes. Set leftover cooking water aside.
• In blender or food processor, purée until smooth, adding leftover cooking water if needed.
• Pour into ice cube trays and freeze.

Yield: 6 cubes

1/4 banana, skin removed
1 tbsp breast milk or formula
   (approx)

• In bowl, mash banana with fork to remove lumps. Add breast milk or formula (if needed) to make banana more appealing for younger babies. Serve immediately to prevent banana from turning brown. Once mashed, banana should not be frozen.

Yield: 1 serving

43

APPLES

When choosing apples, remember the sweeter the better; try Golden Delicious or Fuji.

6 medium apples, washed,
    peeled, cored and quartered

• In steamer, steam apples over boiling water for 10 minutes. Set leftover cooking water aside.
• In blender or food processor, purée until smooth. For very young babies you may choose to add leftover cooking water to thin out the purée. When thinning, add 1 tbsp of liquid at a time.
• Pour into ice cube trays and freeze.

Yield: 10 to 12 cubes

WATERMELON CEREAL

If you are using a watermelon with seeds, strain the watermelon juice through a sieve to remove the seeds before adding infant cereal.

I cup seedless watermelon,
    skinned and cubed
I/4 to I/2 cup iron-fortified rice
    cereal

• Place watermelon in a bowl and purée with handheld immersion blender or regular blender.
• Slowly add rice cereal to watermelon juice and mix until desired consistency is reached.

Yield: 6 to 8 cubes

During the period of 6 to 9 months you need to increase the amount of iron-fortified infant cereal your baby is eating to about 4 to 8 tbsp (60 to 125 ml) per day. If your baby doesn't eat meat, strive for at least 8 tbsp (125 ml) of iron-fortified infant cereal per day (on average) by 9 months. Between 9 to 12 months your baby should be eating about 1/2 cup (125 ml) or more per day.

PEARS

6 medium pears, washed, peeled, cored and quartered

• In steamer, steam pears over boiling water for 8 minutes.
• In blender or food processor, purée until smooth, adding left-over cooking water if needed.
• Pour into ice cube trays and freeze.

Yield: 10 to 12 cubes

PEAS PLEASE

This purée can be made with either fresh or frozen peas.

2 cups frozen peas
3/4 cup leftover cooking water (approx)

• Steam peas over boiling water until tender, about 7 minutes. It may take a little longer if using fresh peas.
• In food processor or with handheld immersion blender, purée peas, adding water as needed, until smooth. Let cool.
• Pour into ice cube trays and freeze.

Yield: 10 cubes

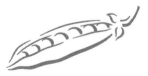

FROM SIX TO NINE MONTHS

45

MASHED AVOCADO

Avocados are one of the few fruits that contain the essential monounsaturated fats. They are rich in potassium and also contain vitamins B, C and E. Introduce avocados early so your baby will learn to love them.

I avocado, washed
I tbsp breast milk or formula
(approx)

• Cut avocado in half. Remove pit and scoop out flesh.
• In bowl, mash avocado with fork, removing lumps. If mixture seems too thick, add milk as needed. Serve immediately to prevent avocado from turning brown. Leftover avocado can be frozen in ice cube trays.

• *To serve:* Defrost and serve at room temperature.

Yield: 3 to 4 cubes

MANGO MASH

Although you can use any type of mango, Filipino mangoes are best because they are sweeter in flavor.

2 Filipino mangoes, washed, skinned and pit removed

• In food processor, purée mangoes until desired consistency is reached.
• If the purée seems too thick, add water a tablespoon at a time until desired consistency is reached.

Yield: 8 to 10 cubes

CUCUMBER

This purée does not need to be warmed and is rather refreshing on a warm day. If you find it too runny, you can always add a little iron fortified infant cereal to thicken it up.

I English cucumber, washed,
   peeled and seeded

• Place cucumber in a bowl and purée with handheld immersion blender. If you do not have an immersion blender, use a food processor or blender.
• Pour into ice cube trays and freeze.

Yield: 6 cubes

MELON

By the time a healthy, full-term infant turns 6 months, there is no need to sterilize the tap water used for the preparation of her baby food.

I medium cantaloupe or
   honeydew melon, washed

• Cut melon in half, remove seeds and scoop out fruit.
• In blender or food processor, purée melon until desired consistency is reached. Add a little tap water a tbsp at a time if needed to smooth out the purée.
• Pour into ice cube trays and freeze.

Yield: 6 to 8 cubes

PEACHES

This purée can also be made with nectarines, plums or apricots.

4 peaches, washed

• In pot of boiling water, plunge peaches for 2 minutes. Remove from water and allow to cool.
• Slit skin with a knife and peel. Cut peach into quarters and remove pit. In steamer, steam fruit over boiling water for 4 minutes.
• In blender or food processor, purée until smooth.
• Pour into ice cube trays and freeze.

Yield: 8 to 10 cubes

BABY BUNNY'S PURÉE

This tasty concoction will have your little bunny wanting more.

3 carrots, washed, peeled and
    sliced
3 parsnips, washed, peeled and
    sliced
1/4 cup Vegetable Stock (2 to 3
    cubes) (recipe, page 58)
or
leftover cooking water (optional)

• In steamer, cook vegetables over boiling water for 15 minutes.
• In blender or food processor, purée until smooth, adding stock (if needed) to achieve desired consistency.
• Pour into ice cube trays and freeze.

Yield: 8 to 10 cubes

SPAGHETTI SQUASH SMASH

1 spaghetti squash

• Using the tip of a knife, pierce squash in 4 places.
• In microwave, cook squash on high until cooked through, about 12 minutes, depending on the size of your squash.
• Cut squash in half lengthwise. Using a large spoon, gently scrape out seeds and discard.
• Using fork, scrape spaghetti-like strands of squash into a bowl. Older babies can eat the squash as is. For younger babies you may choose to purée the squash, adding a little tap water if needed.
• Pour into ice cube trays and freeze.

Yield: 14 cubes

PAPAYA

Papaya mixes well with banana. To prepare, defrost 1 cube of papaya and mix with 1/4 mashed banana. Adding 1 tbsp of milk (breast or formula) will help to thin out the purée, making it more palatable for baby. Serve at room temperature.

I medium papaya, washed

• Cut papaya in half, remove seeds and scoop out fruit.
• In blender or food processor, purée papaya until smooth.
• Pour into ice cube trays and freeze.

Yield: 6 cubes

GO ORANGE!

Canada's new food guide recommends that all Canadians over the age of 2 eat at least one orange vegetable per day. These vegetables are rich in carotenoids, which the body converts to vitamin A. Vitamin A is crucial for maintaining healthy eyes, helps the body fight infection and boosts immune function. Because it's never too early to promote healthy habits, encourage your baby to enjoy a wide variety of orange-colored vegetables. Try Luscious Yams (page 4I), Carrot Apple Delight (page 52), Butternut Squash (page 42) and Spaghetti Squash Smash (page 48). Some orange-colored fruits are also a good source of carotenoids, and they can be eaten in place of an orange vegetable. Such fruits include mango, apricot, papaya and cantaloupe. While oranges are an excellent source of vitamin C and folate, they are not a good source of carotenoids and therefore are not recommended as a replacement for orange vegetables.

SHOULD YOU USE THE MICROWAVE FOR BABY FOOD PREPARATION?

There has been recent controversy over the use of microwaves for food preparation. Concerns have been raised over the potential of microwaves to alter the composition of breast milk, to destroy valuable nutrients in food and to possibly leach toxins from cooking containers. We advise that the microwave never be used to heat baby milk (breast milk or formula) or to warm baby food, in order to avoid dangerous hot spots and the possible disruption of breast milk antibodies.

FRUIT TRIO

This recipe can be made with any combination of either the fruit purées or mashed banana. Experiment to find out which combinations your baby most enjoys!

I cube pear purée
I cube apple purée
I cube cantaloupe purée

• Defrost fruit cubes, mix in bowl and serve at room temperature.

Yield: 1 serving

FRUIT CEREAL

On a hot summer's day, mash frozen apple cubes with equal parts baby cereal and serve when thawed but still cool.

I cube fruit purée (apple or pear
  is ideal to start with)
I tbsp single-grain baby cereal
  (start with rice)
2 tbsp breast milk or formula
  (approx)

• Defrost fruit purée.
• Combine rice with breast milk or formula to make baby rice.
• In saucepan mix rice and fruit together and warm. If combination seems too thick, add extra milk as needed.

Yield: 1 serving

CINNAMON APPLES

Once your baby is comfortable eating a variety of fruit purées, you may want to try a little spice. Cinnamon, a delicious addition to both apple and pear, is a good one to start with. Remember to add the cinnamon before you steam the fruit.

6 medium apples, washed,
  peeled, cored and quartered
I/4 tsp cinnamon

• Sprinkle cinnamon on apples. In steamer, steam over boiling water for 10 minutes.
• In a blender or food processor, purée to desired consistency.
• Pour into ice cube trays and freeze.

Yield: 10 to 12 cubes

51

SWEETEN UP THE DEAL!

If your baby rejects a vegetable, don't get discouraged. Mixing the vegetable with a favorite fruit may make it more appealing. Carrots, for example, mix well with either pear or apple. As your baby becomes more comfortable with the new vegetable, decrease the proportion of fruit and increase the vegetable. Be flexible and experiment to find out which combinations your baby most enjoys.

CARROT APPLE DELIGHT

2 cubes apple purée
I cube carrot purée

• Defrost the purées. In bowl, mix thoroughly and serve at room temperature.

Yield: 1 serving

PEACH BANANA MASH

This recipe can be made with any freshly mashed fruit. If you don't have a peach try a nectarine, pear or papaya.

I/4 banana, skin removed
I/2 peach, washed and skin
  removed
I tbsp breast milk or formula
  (optional)

• In a small bowl, mash banana and peach with fork until desired consistency is reached.
• Add milk if needed and mix thoroughly.
• Serve immediately to prevent fruit from browning.

Yield: 1 serving

BROCCOLI

This purée can be made with either broccoli or cauliflower. As broccoli has a rather strong taste, try combining it with yam when introducing it for the first time. To make, defrost 1 cube yam purée and 1 cube broccoli purée. In bowl, mix and serve at room temperature.

I bunch broccoli, washed and cut
  in florets

• In steamer, cook over boiling water until tender, 10 to 15 minutes. Set leftover cooking water aside.
• In blender or food processor, purée until smooth, adding leftover cooking water if needed.
• Pour into ice cube trays and freeze.

Yield: 10 to 12 cubes

BROCCOLI FIGHTS CANCER

Broccoli, rich in both calcium and iron, also contains phytochemicals known as isothiocyanates. These isothiocyanates have been shown to retard cancer cell growth in research studies. This may explain why people who eat broccoli regularly tend to have a lower risk of colon cancer. Whether these benefits extend to babies and children is not yet known. As colon cancer is the third most common cancer in North America, broccoli is an excellent investment in your baby's future. Introduce it early and serve it frequently.

FROM SIX TO NINE MONTHS

POTATO

Because of their texture, potatoes mix very well with other vegetables. Try them combined with a cube of either broccoli or green bean purée.

I potato, washed, peeled and
    blemishes removed
I/2 cup breast milk or formula

• In saucepan of boiling water, cook potato until tender, about 20 minutes. (Boiling is quicker and often more convenient than baking; however, baking preserves more of the potato's nutrients. To bake, prick skin with fork and place in oven at 400°F for 1 hour. To microwave, prick skin with fork and microwave on high for 4 to 6 minutes).
• In bowl, mash cooked potato with fork, or in blender or food processor, purée. Add milk to achieve desired consistency.
• Pour into ice cube trays and freeze.

Yield: 6 cubes

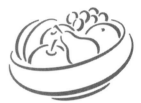

BABY'S FIRST FRUIT SALAD

I/4 small papaya, washed, both
    skin and seeds removed
I/4 avocado, washed and skin
    removed
I tbsp breast milk or formula
(approx)

• In small bowl, mash avocado and papaya together with fork. If mixture seems too thick, add milk to achieve desired consistency.

Yield: 1 serving

GO GREEN!

Health Canada's new food guide recommends that all Canadians over the age of 2 eat at least one dark green vegetable per day. Dark green vegetables are an excellent source of folate, which is needed for the successful division of rapidly dividing cells. Because your baby goes through a period of rapid growth in the first year, tripling his birth weight, it only makes sense to encourage this healthy habit.

Babies under a year have a relatively good acceptance of new foods. However, as children move through the toddler years, many will develop finicky habits. The easiest way, then, to establish a love for green veggies is to introduce them early and serve them frequently. Serve Kale and Apple Purée (page 55); Broccoli, Watercress and Potato (page 63); Green Beans (page 43); Calcium Crunch (page 64) and Peas Please (page 45) as part of your baby's regular meal plan.

KALE AND APPLE PURÉE

4 cups kale, washed, ribs removed
    and chopped
4 apples, washed, peeled, cored
    and quartered
2 tbsp leftover cooking water

• In steamer over boiling water, cook apples and kale until kale is tender, 15 minutes (approx). Set leftover cooking water aside.
• In blender or food processor, purée kale and apples with 2 tbsp leftover cooking water until desired consistency is reached. Add extra cooking water if needed.
• Pour into ice cube trays and freeze.

Yield: 10 cubes

DOWN UNDER FRUIT SALAD

1/3 banana, skin removed

1 slice of papaya, washed, skin and
   seeds removed

1/4 kiwi fruit, washed and skin
   removed

1 tbsp unsweetened apple juice
   (approx)

• In a bowl, mash banana and papaya with fork. Push kiwi through fine sieve to remove seeds; mix with banana and papaya.
• Mix fruit with apple juice as needed. Serve immediately, before banana turns brown.

Yield: 1 serving

BLUEBERRY PURÉE

When blueberries are in season, opt for fresh berries for this recipe; otherwise choose frozen. Frozen fruits and vegetables are picked at their peak and frozen with hours of picking, so they can be a good alternative to fresh.

2 cups blueberries, washed

• In a saucepan, simmer blueberries over low heat, stirring occasionally, for 15 minutes.
• Using handheld immersion blender, purée blueberries until desired consistency is reached. If you do not have an immersion blender, a food processor works well.
• Pour into ice cube trays and freeze.

Yield: 8 cubes

BLUEBERRY BANANA MASH

1/3 banana, skin removed
2 tbsp blueberries, washed
1 tbsp breast milk or formula
(optional)

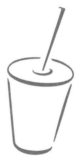

- In a small bowl, mash banana and blueberries with fork until desired consistency is reached.
- Add milk if needed and mix thoroughly.
- Serve immediately to prevent banana from turning brown.

Yield: 1 serving

BERRY BOOST

Packed full of vitamin C and disease-fighting antioxidants, blueberries are a nutritional powerhouse. Antioxidants help to neutralize free radicals, which are the natural bi-product of metabolism. Free radical damage can lead to a variety of life-threatening conditions, including cancer and cardiovascular disease. Get your baby off to a healthy start by serving berries as part of her regular meal plan. Mix blueberry purée into iron-fortified infant cereal or, after 9 months, into full-fat plain yogurt. Ounce per ounce, berries contain more antioxidants than most other fruits and vegetables.

VEGETABLE STOCK

Vegetable stock can be used instead of the leftover cooking water to thin out purées. The following recipes call for vegetable stock; however, its use is optional, as leftover cooking water can be substituted with adequate results. Stock enhances both the taste and nutritional value of the dish.

I leek, trimmed, washed thoroughly (sections separated) and sliced

I parsnip, washed, peeled and sliced

4 stalks celery including leaves, washed, trimmed and sliced

4 carrots, washed, peeled and sliced

I potato, washed, peeled and cut in cubes

I onion, cut in chunks

2 sprigs fresh parsley

I bay leaf

I sprig fresh rosemary

IO cups water

4 peppercorns

• In large pot of water, place vegetables, herbs and peppercorns; bring to a rapid boil. Turn down heat and simmer, partially covered, until vegetables have released their flavor, about 3 to 4 hours.

• Strain and discard vegetables.

• Pour stock into ice cube trays and freeze.

Yield: 32 cubes

FROM SIX TO NINE MONTHS

VEGETABLE RICE

When making this recipe for the first time, start with either carrot or sweet potato.

I cube vegetable purée
I tbsp single-grain baby cereal
(start with rice)
2 tbsp breast milk or formula
(approx)

• Defrost vegetable purée.
• Combine rice with 2 tbsp breast milk or formula to make baby rice.
• In saucepan, mix rice and vegetables together and warm over low heat. If combination seems too thick, add extra milk as needed.

Yield: 1 serving

FLORIDA BREAKFAST

I cube pear purée
I/4 banana, skin removed
I tbsp breast milk or formula
(approx)

• Defrost pear purée.
• In a small bowl, mash banana with fork; mix with pear and milk. Serve immediately to prevent banana from turning brown.

Yield: 1 serving

GROWTH AND DEVELOPMENT

Growth patterns of babies vary depending on multiple factors, such as genetic endowment, gestational age at birth, activity level and race. They also differ in the timing of individual growth spurts. Serial measurements of height, weight and head circumference are much more indicative of growth pattern than is a single measurement. Plot your baby's height, weight and head circumference on a standardized graph (see Appendix III, page 195). Provided your baby is following a smooth growth curve and is thriving, growth is likely occurring at your baby's own pace. Here are some approximate measurements:

RULES OF THUMB FOR GROWTH

WEIGHT, HEIGHT AND HEAD CIRCUMFERENCE

WEIGHT

Weight loss in first few days of life:	5 to 10% of birth weight
Return to birth weight:	7 to 10 days of life
Double birth weight:	4 to 5 months
Average birth weight:	3.5 kg (7.7 lbs)
Average weight at 1 year:	10 kg (22 lbs)
Average weight at 5 years:	20 kg (44 lbs)

HEIGHT

Average length at birth:	50 cm (19.7 inches)
Average height at 3 years:	90 cm (35.4 inches)
Average height at 4 years:	100 cm (39.3 inches), double birth length

HEAD CIRCUMFERENCE

Average head circumference at birth: 35 cm (13.8 inches)
Average head circumference increase: 2 cm (0.8 inch) per month for the first 3 months, then 1 cm (0.4 inch) per month from 4 to 12 months

VEGETABLE TRIO

I potato, washed, peeled and cut
    in cubes
I carrot, washed, peeled and
    sliced
1/4 bunch broccoli, washed and
    cut in florets
1/4 cup Vegetable Stock (2 to 3
    cubes) (recipe, page 58)
or
leftover cooking water (optional)

OKANAGAN SUMMER
SALAD

1/4 peach, washed, pit and skin
    removed (see Peaches recipe,
    page 47)
1/4 pear, washed, cored and skin
    removed
1/2 banana, skin removed
I tbsp breast milk or formula
(approx)

• In small bowl, mash peach,
pear and banana with fork. Add
1 tbsp of milk and mix thoroughly. If mixture seems too
thick, add more milk as needed.

Yield: 1 serving

• In saucepan of boiling water,
cook potato until tender, about
20 minutes.
• In steamer, steam remaining
vegetables until tender, about
15 minutes.
• In blender or food processor,
purée vegetables, adding stock
(if needed) to achieve desired
consistency.
• Pour into ice cube trays and
freeze.

Yield: 12 to 14 cubes

PROCEED WITH CAUTION

The following foods should be delayed for various reasons:

SAFE PREPARATION OF FIRST FOODS

FOOD	RECOMMENDATIONS FOR SERVING
Grapes, Raw carrots, Wieners, Sausages, Cherry tomatoes	To prevent choking, serve finely sliced lengthways. Do not serve in circular pieces.
Honey	Do not serve until I year of age to avoid the risk of botulism. Honey may contain botulism spores, which cannot be killed by the immature gastrointestinal tract.
Whole milk	Do not serve until 12 months of age. Dairy products such as yogurt and cheese may be introduced around 9 months.
Skim, I% and 2% milk	Do not serve until at least 2 years of age, after consultation with your doctor.
Popcorn, Hard candies, Chewing gum, Nuts, Peanuts, Olives, Hard raw veggies like carrots, Raisins, Globs of peanut butter, Ice cubes, Chips, Whole marshmallows, Jellybeans	To prevent choking, avoid until 4 years of age.

WHAT ABOUT NITRATES?

At one time it was recommended that home-prepared carrots, spinach, turnip and beets not be fed to very young infants. The level of nitrates, compared to that in commercially processed vegetables (which removes some nitrates), could be detrimental to the infant kidney. However, now that it is customary to introduce solids at the later age of 6 months, current recommendations do not advise restricting these nutritious vegetables. Nitrates are not a concern for healthy term infants over 4 months of age.

BROCCOLI, WATERCRESS AND POTATO

1/3 bunch broccoli, washed and
    cut in florets
1 potato, washed and baked
2 handfuls fresh watercress, thor-
    oughly washed, stalks removed
1/4 cup Vegetable Stock (2 to 3
    cubes) (recipe, page 58)
or
leftover cooking water (optional)

- Peel potato and cut in cubes.
- In steamer, cook broccoli over boiling water until tender, about 15 minutes; add watercress for last 3 minutes of cooking time.
- In blender or food processor, purée potato and broccoli mixture until smooth, adding stock (if needed) to achieve desired consistency.
- Pour into ice cube trays and freeze.

Yield: 10 to 12 cubes

CALCIUM CRUNCH

I potato, washed and baked
1/3 bunch broccoli, washed and
cut in florets
4 bunches baby bok choy, outer
layers removed, trimmed and
washed between leaves

- Peel potato and cut in chunks.
- In steamer, cook broccoli over boiling water until tender, about 15 minutes. Remove broccoli. Place bok choy in steamer; steam until tender, 4 to 5 minutes. Set aside leftover cooking water.
- Place vegetables in food processor and purée until smooth. If purée seems too thick, add leftover cooking water as needed, 1 tbsp at a time.
- Pour into ice cube trays and freeze.

Yield: 14 to 16 cubes

VEGGIE DELIGHT

I potato, washed, peeled and cut
in cubes
I zucchini, washed, trimmed and
sliced
1/4 bunch broccoli, washed and
cut in florets
1/3 cup Vegetable Stock (3 to 4
cubes) (recipe, page 58)
or
leftover cooking water (optional)

- In saucepan of boiling water, cook potato until tender, about 20 minutes.
- In steamer, cook zucchini and broccoli over boiling water until tender, about 15 minutes.
- In blender or food processor, purée vegetables until smooth, adding vegetable stock or leftover cooking water, if needed, to achieve desired consistency.
- Pour into ice cube trays and freeze.

Yield: 10 to 12 cubes

HOW MUCH CALCIUM?

Ninety-nine percent of the body's skeleton is made up of calcium. During rapid growth in the first 2 years of life it is essential to provide your baby with sufficient calcium to optimize growth potential and to build strong bones. Despite high breast milk or infant formula intake over this period, some babies fail to meet recommended daily intakes of calcium. Furthermore, recommended intakes of calcium increase significantly throughout the first 2 years to reflect the increasing demands of growth. To increase your baby's calcium levels, offer vegetables naturally high in calcium such as bok choy, broccoli and watercress.

OPTIMAL CALCIUM REQUIREMENTS

AGE	RECOMMENDED CALCIUM INTAKE
0-6 mths	210 mg/day
6-12 mths	270 mg/day
1-3 yrs	500 mg/day
4-8 yrs	800 mg/day
9-18 yrs	1500 mg/day
Pregnancy or breastfeeding	
18 and younger	1300 mg/day
19-50 yrs	1000 mg/day

CALCIUM CONTENT OF SELECTED FOODS

FOOD	SERVING	CALCIUM (mg)
Milk	250 ml (1 cup)	315
Firm cheese	50 g (1.6 oz)	350
Yogurt	125 ml (1/2 cup)	196
Baked beans	250 ml (1 cup)	163
Bok choy, cooked	125 ml (1/2 cup)	84
Broccoli, cooked	125 ml (1/2 cup)	38
Chickpeas, cooked	250 ml (1 cup)	84
Orange	1 medium	52
Rhubarb, cooked	125 ml (1/2 cup)	184
Salmon, canned	1/2 213-g can (7oz)	225
Sardines, canned	1/2 213-g can (7oz)	210

Source: Standing Committee on the Scientific Evaluation of Dietary Reference Intakes, Food and Nutrition Board, Institute of Medicine, 1997.

RETHINKING FAT FOR BABIES

In today's health-conscious society adults place great emphasis on reducing fat and cholesterol intake in an effort to prevent heart disease and control weight. Such restrictions, however, can be dangerous when applied to infants under 2 years of age. During this time of rapid growth, fats are used as a dense source of calories for energy and constitute a major part of the developing brain. Unlike with adults, there is no evidence that restricting fats in babies prevents disease later in life. For this reason, the Canadian Paediatric Society recommends that fats constitute approximately 50 percent of the infant's diet until the age of 2. The majority of this fat is obtained from breast milk or infant formula, followed by milk. As your child grows, the need for fats diminishes and lower-fat choices may be appropriate. Until 2 years, however, baby needs whole-fat dairy products. Do not place your baby on a low-fat diet unless advised by your doctor.

VICHYSSOISE

2 large potatoes, washed, peeled and cut in cubes
1 1/2 leeks, trimmed, washed thoroughly (sections separated) and sliced
2 cups Salt-Free Chicken Stock (approx) (recipe, page 76)
1/4 cup chopped fresh parsley (optional)

• In large saucepan, pour chicken stock over leeks and potatoes, ensuring there is enough stock to cover the vegetables. Bring to a rapid boil. Reduce heat and simmer, partially covered, until tender, 30 minutes, stirring occasionally.
• Remove from heat, add parsley (if using) and stir.
• With a slotted spoon remove vegetables and place in blender or food processor; set leftover stock aside.
• Purée, adding leftover stock as needed, until desired consistency is reached.
• Pour into ice cube trays and freeze.

Yield: 20 to 22 cubes

TEETHING

At approximately 6 to 7 months of age most babies will cut their first tooth. However, some babies are born with teeth and some do not cut their first tooth until over 1 year of age. Teething may cause drooling, irritability, increased bowel movements and a reluctance to eat solid foods. Teething does not cause fever. For babies 3 months or younger, immediately contact your doctor in the event of fever of 100.4°F or greater. To alleviate symptoms of teething, offer your baby something firm to chew on, such as a chilled teething ring. To prevent a painful rash from drooling, use petroleum jelly as a barrier. Offer soft foods but do not force meals, and increase the number of breast milk or formula feedings to alleviate hunger. For continued teething discomfort, use pain-relieving medicine as advised by your doctor. Teeth cleaning should begin with the appearance of the first tooth and should take place twice a day, as well as after sweeter foods such as dried fruit. Start teeth cleaning using a damp washcloth, and switch to a baby toothbrush with a smear of toothpaste as more teeth appear.

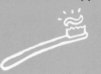

TIME OF ERUPTION OF PRIMARY TEETH

TOOTH TYPE	MONTHS	
	UPPER	LOWER
Front teeth	6 +/- 2	7 +/- 2
Front side teeth	9 +/- 2	7 +/- 2
First molars	14 +/- 4	12 +/- 4
Canines	18 +/- 2	16 +/- 2
Second molars	24 +/- 4	20 +/- 4

Reprinted from *Nelson Essentials of Paediatrics*, 4th edition, Behrman R. and Kliegman R., page 488. W. B. Saunders Company, Philadelphia, PA. Copyright 2002, with permission from Elsevier.

VEGETABLE STEW

4 cups Vegetable Stock (not optional) (recipe, page 58)

2 carrots, washed, trimmed, peeled and sliced

I parsnip, washed, trimmed, peeled and sliced

2 stalks celery, washed, trimmed and sliced

I potato, washed, peeled and cut in cubes

I zucchini, washed, trimmed and sliced

I cup broccoli florets, washed

1/2 leek, trimmed, washed thoroughly (sections separated) and sliced

1/4 cup chopped fresh parsley (optional)

• In large saucepan, combine stock and vegetables. Bring to a boil. Reduce heat and simmer, partially covered, for 30 minutes, stirring occasionally.

• Add parsley (if using) and continue to simmer for another 5 minutes. If there seems to be too much liquid, remove the lid for the last 5 to 10 minutes of cooking time. This will allow the liquid to evaporate and the flavors to concentrate.

• Once stew is thick, pour contents through a strainer, separating vegetables from stock; set stock aside.

• In blender or food processor, purée vegetables to desired consistency. Over low heat, slowly mix vegetables and stock together, and continue to simmer for another 5 to 10 minutes. When done, stew should be the consistency of a thick soup.

• Pour into ice cube trays and freeze.

Yield: 26 cubes

BROWN RICE AND VEGETABLES

2 cups Salt-Free Chicken Stock
(recipe, page 76)
I cup broccoli florets, washed
2 carrots, washed, peeled and cut
in sticks
I/3 cup whole-grain brown rice

• In saucepan, bring stock to boil. Add broccoli and carrots; reduce heat and simmer with lid on to prevent evaporation of stock.
• Once tender, drain vegetables; save stock. (Cooking the vegetables in stock preserves nutrients that would otherwise be lost.)
• Pour stock back into saucepan; add rice.
• Bring to a boil, stir once and reduce heat. Cover and simmer for 50 minutes. Remove from heat and allow to stand for 10 minutes.
• In blender or food processor, purée rice, excess stock and vegetables to desired consistency.
• Pour into ice cube trays and freeze.

Yield: 12 to 14 cubes

BROCCOLI AND SWEET POTATO PURÉE

2 sweet potatoes, washed,
peeled and blemishes
removed
I I/2 cups broccoli florets, washed

• Cut sweet potatoes into cubes.
• In saucepan of water, simmer potatoes until tender, 20 to 30 minutes. Remove from water; set leftover cooking water aside.
• Using steamer, steam broccoli over boiling water for 10 minutes.
• In blender or food processor, purée broccoli and potatoes. Add leftover cooking water to achieve desired consistency.
• Pour into ice cube trays and freeze.

Yield: 14 to 16 cubes

RATATOUILLE

This dish is also tasty served with cheese (after 9 months). To prepare, defrost 2 cubes and mix in a saucepan over low heat with 1 tbsp of grated mozzarella cheese.

I can (14 oz) chopped tomatoes

I cup water

I potato, washed, peeled and cut in cubes

I cup broccoli florets, washed

I zucchini, washed, trimmed and sliced

I red pepper, washed, peeled with potato peeler and diced

10 green beans, washed, trimmed, stringy bits removed, and diced

1/3 cup chopped fresh basil (optional)

• In large saucepan, mix tomatoes and water; add vegetables and bring to a boil. Reduce heat and simmer partially covered for 30 minutes, stirring occasionally. When done, ratatouille should be the consistency of a thick stew. If there is too much liquid, remove the lid for the last 5 to 10 minutes of cooking time. (This allows the flavors to concentrate and the liquid to evaporate.)

• Remove from heat, add basil (if using) and stir.

• With a slotted spoon, remove vegetables and place in blender or food processor. Set leftover cooking juices aside. Purée, adding juices as needed.

• Pour into ice cube trays and freeze.

Yield: 20 to 22 cubes

STRAWBERRY STEW

Because strawberries can be difficult to digest, introduce them once other fruits and vegetables are well established. Serving them on their own will help you identify any reactions your baby may have. This recipe can be made with fresh or frozen berries.

I lb strawberries, washed, hulled

• In a saucepan, cook berries on medium heat for 15 minutes.
• Push through sieve to remove seeds.
• Pour into ice cube trays and freeze.

Yield: 8 cubes

ROASTED VEGGIE MASH

I potato, washed and peeled
4 small beets, washed and peeled
I carrot, washed, trimmed and
    peeled
I parsnip, washed, trimmed and
    peeled
3 tbsp olive oil
I/3 cup breast milk or formula
    (approx)

• Cut potato, beets, carrot and parsnip into cubes. In bowl, toss with 2 tbsp olive oil.
• In roasting pan, bake vegetables in 350°F oven until tender, about 50 minutes.
• For a nice lumpy texture, mash with potato masher or fork, adding 1 tbsp olive oil and milk as needed (or if desired, use blender or food processor to purée until smooth).
• Pour into ice cube trays and freeze.

Yield: 12 to 14 cubes

DRIED FRUIT PURÉE

The flavor of this purée is quite rich. At around 9 months babies can eat it mixed with cottage cheese or yogurt to make it more palatable.

10 pitted dried apricots

15 pitted dried prunes

1 1/2 cups water

2 medium apples, washed, peeled
  and quartered

1 cup water (for thinning)

• In a saucepan, cover dried apricots and prunes with water; bring to a boil. Reduce heat and simmer, partially covered, for 15 minutes.

• Add apples and stir; continue to simmer for another 10 minutes. Remove from heat.

• In blender or food processor, purée mixture (adding more water if necessary) until smooth.

• Pour into ice cube trays and freeze.

Yield: 8 to 10 cubes

BABY'S BACKED UP!

There is a wide range of normal bowel patterns for infants and toddlers, from several daily bowel movements to only one bowel movement every few days. A slowing of the normal pattern for your baby does not necessarily indicate constipation. Grunting, groaning and a red face are all normal displays during stooling and are not an expression of pain. True constipation, on the other hand, is the passing of very hard, painful stools (associated with crying) and is quite rare in infancy. Weaning from breast milk to formula, and changing brands or type of formula are the most common reasons for an alteration in the nature or frequency of stool. Often, a change in the bowel pattern causes more concern for the parent than it does for the baby. Unlike an adult, baby is not aware or distressed by the infrequency of bowel movements. A temporary increase of fiber in the diet will likely alleviate it; try Dried Fruit Purée (recipe, page 72). Contact your doctor if your baby has symptoms of true constipation or if you notice blood in the stool or fever. Don't administer a medicinal laxative to your infant; these can be harmful if used without a doctor's supervision.

Chicken

Once your baby has tried a number of fruits and vegetables you can begin mixing them with chicken to make the variety of interesting recipes found in this book. Chicken is an excellent source of energy and protein, which is needed for muscle development, as well as for building and repairing bodily tissue. Chicken is also a source of omega-6 fatty acids, which are essential for brain growth and development. Poaching is the ideal method of cooking chicken for a baby. See page 36 for a poached chicken recipe.

74

CHICKEN AND YAMS

1 large yam, washed, peeled and
   cubed
1 recipe Poached Chicken Breast
   (page 36)
1/4 cup leftover poaching water

• In steamer, steam yam over boiling water until tender, about 20 minutes.
• Chop chicken. In blender or food processor, purée chicken, yam and poaching water. If purée seems too thick, add extra water to achieve desired consistency.
• Pour into ice cube trays and freeze.

Yield: 14 cubes

CHICKEN APPLE DELIGHT

2 apples, washed, peeled and
   quartered
1 recipe Poached Chicken Breast
   (page 36)
2 tbsp unsweetened apple juice
   (approx)

• In steamer, steam apples over boiling water for 10 minutes.
• In blender or food processor, purée chicken, apples and unsweetened apple juice to achieve desired consistency. If the purée seems too thick, add a little more apple juice as needed.
• Pour into ice cube trays and freeze.

Yield: 10 cubes

SALMONELLA

Salmonella is a bacterial infection of the gastrointestinal tract that affects both children and adults, but, most commonly, infants between 2 and 6 months of age. Sources of infection can be contaminated water, poultry, beef, eggs and milk. It may also be transmitted by infected household pets or other persons. The incubation period is 6 to 72 hours. There is usually an abrupt onset of diarrhea (which may contain blood), vomiting and fever, which may last 2 to 5 days. Symptoms may become severe, particularly in young infants. It is important to contact your doctor if you suspect salmonella. There is usually no antibiotic treatment necessary, but your baby must be monitored to prevent dehydration.

It is very important to prevent contamination of food and utensils by carefully cleaning all surfaces, utensils and refrigerator shelves that have come in contact with raw or partially cooked meat. All meat and eggs should be well cooked before serving, and never serve unpasteurized milk or unpasteurized apple juice. Unlike adults, infants and children have an additional risk of infection from contact with contaminated soil or debris left by pets or shoes. Data suggests this contamination plays an even greater role in infection of children than does contaminated food. To minimize this risk, remove shoes indoors and keep floors clean.

SALT-FREE CHICKEN STOCK

Chicken stock, which can easily be made in bulk and frozen, can be used to thin out purées. However, if you do not have the time to make stock, do not let this stop you from preparing homemade chicken for your baby. Many specialty stores now carry salt-free chicken stock. (Avoid using commercial chicken stocks, as they are often high in added salt.) Leftover poaching water can be substituted with adequate results. Stock is best, however, as it serves to enhance flavor and contains calcium, which leaches from the chicken bones during cooking.

For this recipe, chicken wings are an economical choice, but any cut will do. A leftover carcass makes a good substitute as well.

3 carrots, washed, peeled and
    sliced
3 stalks celery (including leaves),
    washed and sliced
I onion, cut in chunks
I parsnip, washed, peeled and
    sliced
I sprig fresh rosemary
I bay leaf
6 peppercorns
5 chicken wings
10 cups water

• In large pot, combine vegetables, herbs and chicken. Cover with water and bring to a boil. Turn down heat and simmer, partially covered, until chicken and vegetables release their flavor, 3 to 4 hours.
• Strain the mixture into bowl or pitcher; discard both chicken and vegetables.
• Pour stock into ice cube trays and freeze.

Yield: 32 cubes

MAKE USE OF BABY'S LOVE OF THE SWEET

Babies tend to have an innate preference for sweet-tasting foods, and this preference can be used to encourage a taste for different flavors and textures. For example, if your baby rejects a new food, combining it with baby's favorite fruit may make it more appealing. Most of the chicken purées described may be combined with a little applesauce to make a naturally sweeter version.

BABY CHICKEN

2 carrots, washed, peeled and
  sliced
I parsnip, washed, peeled and
  sliced
I recipe Poached Chicken Breast
  (page 36)
1/4 cup Salt-Free Chicken Stock (2
  to 3 cubes) (recipe, page 76)
or
leftover poaching water

• In steamer, steam carrots and parsnip over boiling water until tender, about 10 minutes.
• In blender or food processor, purée chicken, vegetables and stock to achieve desired consistency. If purée seems too thick, add either extra chicken stock or leftover poaching water.
• *Tip:* For a sweeter version try adding unsweetened apple juice instead of stock.
• Pour into ice cube trays and freeze.

Yield: 10 to 12 cubes

CHICKEN AND WINTER VEGETABLES

1/2 potato, washed, peeled and
  cut in cubes
I carrot, washed, peeled and
  sliced
I cup broccoli florets, washed
I recipe Poached Chicken Breast
  (page 36)
1/4 cup Salt-Free Chicken Stock (2
  to 3 cubes) (recipe, page 76)
or
leftover poaching water

• In saucepan of boiling water, cook potato for 20 minutes.
• Using steamer, cook carrot and broccoli over boiling water until tender, about 10 minutes.
• In blender or food processor, purée vegetables and chicken, slowly adding chicken stock to achieve desired consistency.
• Pour into ice cube trays and freeze.

Yield: 10 to 12 cubes

SICILIAN CHICKEN

This dish can also be served with cheese (after age 9 months). To prepare, defrost 3 cubes and mix in saucepan over low heat with 1 tbsp of grated cheddar cheese.

1/4 onion, finely diced

1 tbsp olive oil

2 tomatoes, washed, skinned and seeded (see Skinned Seeded Tomatoes, page 124)

1 tbsp chopped fresh parsley (optional)

1 recipe Poached Chicken Breast (page 36)

1 baked potato, skin removed, chopped

• In frying pan, heat olive oil over low heat; sauté onion until translucent.
• Add tomatoes and parsley (if using); continue to sauté for another 10 minutes.
• In blender or food processor, purée tomatoes, chicken and potato to achieve desired consistency.
• Pour into ice cube trays and freeze.

Yield: 10 to 12 cubes

CHICKEN AND BUTTERNUT SQUASH PURÉE

1 butternut squash, washed and ends removed

1 recipe Poached Chicken Breast (page 36)

1/4 cup Salt-Free Chicken Stock (2 to 3 cubes) (recipe, page 76)

or

leftover poaching water

• Peel squash, cut in half, remove seeds and cut in cubes.
• In steamer, cook squash over boiling water until tender, about 10 to 12 minutes.
• In blender or food processor, purée squash and chicken, adding stock as necessary to achieve desired consistency.
• Pour into ice cube trays and freeze.

Yield: 14 to 16 cubes

79

WHAT ARE TRANS FATS?

A high-fat diet is essential for optimal growth and development in the first 2 years of life. Fat intake ensures proper brain and nerve development and supplies energy for growth. This fat is available in whole foods, most notably breast milk, dairy, meats and oils.

There are four kinds of fats: monounsaturated fat, polyunsaturated fat, saturated fat and trans fat. Monounsaturated fats and polyunsaturated fats are considered good fats. Saturated fats are found in meat, dairy and some vegetables and include butter, shortening, animal fat, palm oil and coconut oil. Trans fats are dangerous fats and contribute to diabetes, heart disease, immune dysfunction and obesity in adults. There is no safe amount of these fats and they have been labeled the biggest food-processing disaster in history. Trans fats are placed in processed foods to prolong shelf life; they have little nutritional value. Packaging and labeling laws do not require that trans fats be identified in the ingredients, so stay away from any foods which list "partially hydrogenated" or trans-fat to be safe. To avoid the risks of these fats eat whole foods and avoid highly processed foods as much as possible.

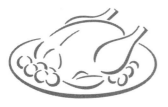

THANKSGIVING DINNER

I medium sweet potato, washed,
   peeled and cubed
I recipe Poached Chicken (or
   Turkey) Breast (page 36)
I/3 cup Salt-Free Chicken Stock
(3 to 4 cubes) (recipe, page 76)
or
leftover poaching water

• In saucepan of boiling water,
cook sweet potato until tender,
20 to 30 minutes; drain.
• Chop chicken. In blender or
food processor, purée chick-
en, sweet potato and stock.
If purée seems too thick, add
either extra stock or leftover
poaching water to achieve
desired consistency.
• Pour into ice cube trays and
freeze.

Yield: 12 to 14 cubes

TURKEY AND SWEET POTATO HASH

For very young babies, you may
choose to purée this dish before
freezing.

2 tbsp canola oil
I/2 lb ground turkey
I medium sweet potato, washed
   and baked
I/2 cup frozen peas
I/2 cup of water

• In frying pan, heat oil over
medium heat. Add turkey and
brown for 10 minutes.
• Cut sweet potato in half,
scoop out flesh and mash with
fork. Add sweet potato to pan
and sauté for 5 minutes.
• Add peas and water. Mix
thoroughly and cook for
another 5 minutes. Let cool.
• Pour into ice cube trays and
freeze.

Yield: 14 cubes

Red Meat

In an effort to minimize the risk of heart disease and stroke, many people now avoid red meat. Others believe that reduced intake of carbohydrates and increased intake of lean meats, including red meat, actually reduces obesity and heart disease in adults. Studies show that cholesterol and animal fat intake during infancy does not contribute to heart disease later in life. Further, iron deficiency is the most common nutritional problem among children and may have serious health consequences. Because red meat is the richest source of iron available, its consumption will benefit your baby. The method of choice for cooking red meat is stewing, as it tenderizes the meat while it cooks.

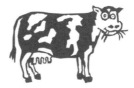

MAMA'S HOMEMADE BEEF STEW

8 cubes stewing beef

2 cups water

2 carrots, washed, trimmed, peeled and sliced

1 potato, washed, peeled and cut in cubes

1/4 onion, cut in half

2 celery stalks, washed, trimmed and sliced

2 chopped fresh sage leaves (optional)

2 sprigs fresh parsley (optional)

• In large pot, bring beef and water to a boil. Add carrots, potato, onion, celery and herbs (if using). Reduce heat and simmer, partially covered, until meat is thoroughly cooked and vegetables are tender, about 25 to 30 minutes. Stir occasionally. The consistency should be that of a thick stew. If there is too much liquid, remove lid for last 5 to 10 minutes of cooking. (This enables the water to evaporate and the flavors to concentrate.)

• With a slotted spoon, place meat and vegetables in blender or food processor. Set leftover cooking juices aside. Purée, adding juices as needed to achieve desired consistency.

• Pour into ice cube trays and freeze.

Yield: 18 to 20 cubes

IRON-DEFICIENCY ANEMIA

Iron is a major component of hemoglobin, which enables red blood cells to transport oxygen throughout the body. Iron deficiency is a common finding among infants, children and teenagers. Risk factors for the development of iron-deficiency anemia include prematurity, low birth weight, anemia in the mother during pregnancy, too early introduction of cow's milk or solid foods, low meat intake, breastfeeding beyond 6 months without other sources of iron, infant formula not supplemented with iron, and some unusual dietary practices.

During the rapid growth period in the first year of life, infants almost triple their blood volume, and their requirement for iron increases from 4 mg per day to 7 mg per day. For this reason Health Canada recommendations advise the introduction of iron-rich foods, including meat and fish, first. These requirements are higher for premature infants. If iron needs are not met, infants may become deficient, which leads to poor weight gain, recurrent illness, poor appetite, gastrointestinal problems, irritability, decreased attention span and decreased physical activity. If the deficiency persists it is possible that cognitive development may be impaired. If iron deficiency is suspected, a blood test can confirm the diagnosis.

To maintain your baby's adequate iron intake be sure her diet includes a wide variety of iron-rich foods such as iron-fortified baby cereals, poultry, red meat, broccoli, spinach and legumes. Continue iron-fortified baby cereals throughout the first 2 years by mixing with other foods and serving often. The amount of iron in infant formula and supplements is often much higher than the recommended daily intake because the amount of iron actually absorbed by the body is quite small. To enhance absorption, serve iron-rich foods with foods high in vitamin C, such as tomatoes, baked potato and citrus fruit.

MAXWELL'S MINTED LAMB

I cup water

I can (I4 oz) diced tomatoes

8 cubes stewing lamb

I potato, washed, peeled and cut
in cubes

2 carrots, washed, peeled and
sliced

2 stalks celery, washed, trimmed
and sliced

1/4 onion, diced

I tbsp chopped fresh mint
(optional)

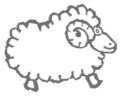

• In saucepan, mix water with tomatoes and add lamb. Bring to a boil.

• Add vegetables; reduce heat and continue to simmer until they are tender, 25 to 30 minutes. Stir occasionally. The consistency should be that of a thick stew. If you feel there is too much liquid, remove the lid for last 5 to 10 minutes of cooking. (This will allow the water to evaporate and flavors to concentrate.)

• Add mint (if using) and stir.

• With a slotted spoon place lamb and vegetables in blender or food processor. Set leftover cooking juices aside.

• Purée, adding juices as needed to achieve desired consistency.

• Pour into ice cube trays and freeze.

Yield: 18 to 20 cubes

SHEPHERD'S MASH

I tbsp olive oil

1/4 onion, diced

I can (14 oz) diced tomatoes

I tbsp chopped fresh parsley
(optional)

I carrot, washed, peeled and
sliced

I clove garlic, mashed (optional)

8 cubes stewing beef

1/4 cup water

2 medium potatoes, washed,
peeled and cut in cubes

• In saucepan, heat oil over medium heat; sauté onion until translucent, about 5 minutes. Stir in tomatoes, parsley, carrot and garlic (if using); continue to sauté for another 5 minutes.
• Add beef and water; bring to a boil. Reduce heat and simmer, partially covered, until meat is thoroughly cooked, 25 to 30 minutes. Stir occasionally.
• Meanwhile, in saucepan of boiling salted water, cook potatoes until tender; drain.

• In blender or food processor, purée meat mixture and potatoes until desired consistency is reached.
• Pour into ice cube trays and freeze.

Yield: 16 to 18 cubes

EASY BEEF HASH

1/2 lb ground beef

I cup canned diced tomatoes

I potato, washed and baked

• Brown beef in nonstick frying pan for 5 minutes, until no longer pink. Add tomatoes and continue to sauté for another 10 minutes, stirring occasionally.
• Meanwhile, cut potato in half, scoop out flesh and mash with fork. Add potato to pan; continue to sauté for 10 minutes.
• Pour into ice cube trays and freeze.
• *Tip:* For very young babies you may choose to purée in a food processor before freezing.

Yield: 12 to 14 cubes

PORK AND APPLE
PURÉE

8 cubes stewing pork

I cup water

4 apples, washed, peeled, cored
   and sectioned

• In saucepan, bring pork and water to a boil. Reduce heat and simmer, partially covered, until pork is thoroughly cooked, 25 to 30 minutes. Set aside and save stewing water.

• In steamer, steam apples over boiling water for 10 minutes.

• In blender or food processor, purée apples and pork to achieve desired consistency. (For younger babies it may be necessary to add leftover stewing water to thin out the purée. When adding liquid, start with 1 tbsp at a time.)

• Pour into ice cube trays and freeze.

Yield: 12 cubes

Although juice is a source of vitamin C, your baby does not need it and there is no nutritional reason to give it to an infant before the age of one. This is due in part to the fact that the Recommended Nutrient Intake for vitamin C for infants (6 to 12 months) is 20 mg per day and this amount is easily obtained by drinking breast milk or infant formula and eating vegetables and fruit.

The problem with juice is that it is all too common to consume too much of it and this can indirectly contribute to inadequate intake of other nutrients. Furthermore, the sorbitol and fructose content of juice can cause diarrhea, poor weight gain and failure to thrive. Excessive juice intake can also lead to dental caries. If offering juice, only serve 100 percent real fruit juice and limit it to 60 to 125 ml (1/4 to 1/2 cup) per day. Serve it in a cup and don't dilute it with water. With diluting comes the tendency to serve it more frequently, which only serves to continually bathe the teeth in plaque-forming bacteria.

MIDDLE-EASTERN
BEEF STEW

2 tbsp olive oil

1/4 onion, diced

I tsp freshly grated ginger
(optional)

I tsp ground cumin (optional)

1/2 medium eggplant, washed,
peeled and diced

I can (19 oz) chickpeas, drained
and rinsed

8 cubes stewing beef

I carrot, washed, peeled and
sliced

2 cups water

1/4 cup chopped fresh parsley
(optional)

• In saucepan, heat oil over medium heat; sauté onion and ginger for 5 minutes. Add cumin, eggplant and chickpeas; continue to sauté for another 20 minutes.

• Add beef, carrot and water; stir. Bring to a boil. Reduce heat and simmer, partially covered, until meat is cooked, 25 to 30 minutes. Stir occasionally. The consistency should be that of a thick stew. If you feel there is too much liquid, remove the lid for last 5 to 10 minutes of cooking. (This will allow the water to evaporate and flavors to concentrate.)

• Remove from heat. Add parsley (if using) and stir.

• With a slotted spoon, place beef, vegetables and chickpeas in blender or food processor. Set leftover cooking juices aside. Purée, adding juices as needed to achieve desired consistency.

• Pour into ice cube trays and freeze.

Yield: 16 to 18 cubes

Fish

Fish is easy to cook, high in protein and one of the few sources of omega-3 fatty acids. Fish is also easy for your baby to chew, whether served on its own or puréed with vegetables. Remember to always look for bones when serving fish. The only way to be sure there are no bones is to allow the fish to cool and then flake it apart with your fingers.

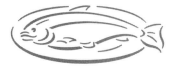

FISH AND PEAR PURÉE

Once your baby has eaten fish on its own, try it mixed with fruit. Because the natural sweetness of fruit appeals to babies, this recipe is likely to be a hit.

6 oz sole fillet

2 pears, washed, peeled, cored and quartered

2 tbsp leftover cooking water (approx)

• In a steamer over boiling water, steam fish and pears until fish is cooked through, about 20 minutes, depending on the thickness of the fish. Set leftover cooking water aside. Allow fish to cool. Flake fish apart with fingers to remove bones.

• Transfer fish and pears to food processor and purée, adding leftover cooking water as needed to achieve desired consistency.

• Pour into ice cube trays and freeze.

Yield: 10 to 12 cubes

WEST COAST SALMON

8 oz salmon fillet

I tbsp chopped fresh dill (optional)

I tbsp finely diced onion

Dash lemon juice

I potato, washed, peeled and cut in cubes

I tbsp breast milk or formula (approx) (3.25% milk after age 12 months)

• Place fish on tinfoil. Coat with dill (if using), onion and dash of lemon juice. Wrap in foil and bake in 375°F oven until thoroughly cooked, about 20 minutes.

• Open foil and allow to cool. Flake fish apart with fingers to remove skin and bones. Set fish aside; save cooking juices.

• In pot of boiling water, cook potato until tender, about 20 minutes. In blender or food processor, purée potato, fish, cooking juices and milk. If mixture seems too thick, add extra milk to achieve desired consistency.

• Fill ice cube trays and freeze.

Yield: 12 cubes

WHAT ARE OMEGA-3 FATTY ACIDS?

Omega-3 fatty acids are highly unsaturated long-chain fatty acids thought to significantly reduce the development of heart disease in adults and to improve cognitive function and vision in infants. It has long been known that Greenland Inuit, Japanese and Scandinavian populations have much lower rates of heart disease. The common feature among these populations is the consumption of fish, in particular cold-water marine fish, such as salmon, trout, tuna and sardines. The substance in oily fish has now been identified as omega-3 fatty acid. Further research has revealed that 40 percent of the polyunsaturated fatty acids that make up the brain and 60 percent of those that make up the retina are a type of omega-3 known as DHA (docosahexaenoic acid).

At one time, humans consumed far higher quantities of omega-3 fatty acids than we do today. This is because prior to the agricultural revolution, humans consumed wild animals that grazed on omega-3 rich plants. Interestingly, human milk contains omega-3 fatty acids at a ratio to other fats similar to that in our ancestors' diet. Today, animals raised for consumption are fed diets such as corn and soybean, which are very low in omega-3. Consequently the ratio of omega-3 to other fats in our diet has been reduced 10 to 30 fold. Omega-3 is present in significant quantities in oily fish, human breast milk, flax seed, omega-3 eggs and, to a lesser extent, in regular eggs. Consequently, for those who do not consume fish, omega-3 levels are far below recommended intakes. To increase intake and reap the benefits of omega-3, adults should consume 2 to 3 servings of fish per week.

91

RED SNAPPER SALSA PROVENÇAL

12 oz red snapper fillet

1/4 red onion, finely diced

2 tomatoes, skinned, seeded and diced (see Skinned Seeded Tomatoes, page 124)

1 tbsp chopped fresh parsley (optional)

1 tbsp chopped fresh basil (optional)

1 potato, baked, skin removed

• Place fish on tinfoil. In bowl mix onion, tomatoes and herbs (if using). Coat fish with this tomato salsa. Wrap fish in foil.

• Bake in 375°F oven until fish is thoroughly cooked, about 25 minutes. Open foil to allow cooling. Flake fish apart with fingers to remove skin and bones.

• In blender or food processor, purée fish, salsa and potato to achieve desired consistency.

• Fill ice cube trays and freeze.

Yield: 14 cubes

CHOOSING SAFE FISH

Concerns about toxins from fish arose in the 1960s following serious fish-related mercury poisonings in Japan. No such incidents have occurred in North America; however, concerns about the level of mercury in fish are valid. The earth's crust and waste discharge from industry are the main sources of mercury absorbed by fish. Once consumed by humans, mercury can accumulate in the body. If mercury reaches toxic levels, the result can be damage to the nervous system.

Nearly all fish have trace levels of mercury that are harmless to humans. Because mercury accumulates in the food chain, larger predatory fish such as fresh and frozen tuna, shark, swordfish, escolar, marlin and orange roughy have higher mercury levels. Health Canada recommends that women who are pregnant or may become pregnant and breastfeeding mothers eat no more than 150 grams of these species per month.

Young children between 5 and 11 years of age can safely eat up to 125 grams per month and very young children between 1 and 4 years of age should eat no more than 75 grams per month. For babies it makes sense to avoid these species.

When feeding your family it is advisable to serve fish that is low in mercury more often. These species include salmon (wild, farmed or canned), shrimp, prawns, rainbow trout, Atlantic mackerel, sole and Dover sole. The following species are considered to have moderate mercury levels: Atlantic cod, bass or white bass, halibut, lake trout, sablefish, black cod or Alaskan black cod and sea bass. Because children under 2 are more susceptible to toxicity, the Ministry of Health for the Province of British Columbia recommends they eat no more than 2 servings of these species per month. These recommendations apply to retail fish only. If you consume sport fish you may want to consult Environment Canada at http://www.ec.gc.ca/mercury/en/fc.cfm for more information.

Health Canada recently revised its position on canned albacore tuna. Because the mercury levels of canned albacore tuna are higher than other species of tuna, Health Canada recommends that women who are pregnant, those who may become pregnant and those who are breast-feeding eat no more than 4 food guide servings (1 serving = 1/2 cup or 75 grams) per week. Very young children between 1 and 4 years old can safely eat up to 1 serving of canned albacore tuna per week and children between 5 and 11 can eat 2 servings per week. These recommendations do not apply to canned light tuna, which has relatively low mercury levels. As babies are more susceptible to toxicity, opt for canned light tuna when possible and aim for no more than 2 servings per month.

A recent study revealed that PCBs and other toxins in farmed salmon are significantly higher than in the wild species. Although the levels of PCBs are well below recommended limits, for now it is advisable to choose wild salmon whenever possible.

In summary, the benefits of fish consumption far outweigh the risks, and a healthy diet should contain at least 2 servings of fish per week.

FISH OIL AND ASTHMA

In addition to having a low incidence of heart disease, populations that regularly consume oily, marine fish also have low incidences of certain inflammatory diseases. Early clinical trials have shown fish oil to be beneficial in diseases such as rheumatoid arthritis, psoriasis, cystic fibrosis and inflammatory bowel disease. The beneficial properties of oily fish are thought to be due to an omega-3 fatty acid known as EPA (eicosapentaenoic acid), which works as a potent anti-inflammatory. This theory has provoked several studies into the benefit of fish oil for asthma, a chronic inflammatory disease of the airway. The most promising result was a study conducted in Australia, showing an almost one-third reduction in the incidence of asthma among children who consumed fresh oily fish more than once a week.

TUNA SALAD

1/4 can (6 oz) light tuna, drained

1 tbsp cucumber, washed, peeled and finely diced

1/4 avocado, washed, skin removed, pitted and mashed

1 tsp chopped fresh cilantro (optional)

• In bowl, combine ingredients and serve.

• *Tip:* For younger babies you may choose to use a blender or food processor to purée to achieve desired consistency.

Yield: 1 serving

SALMON AND VEGETABLES WITH CREAMY DILL SAUCE

10 oz salmon fillet

1 tbsp lemon juice

1 tbsp diced onion (approx)

2 carrots, washed, peeled and chopped

2 cups broccoli florets, washed

1 rounded tsp butter

1 rounded tsp flour

1/3 cup breast milk or formula (3.25% milk after age 12 months)

1 tbsp chopped fresh dill

• Place salmon on tinfoil. Sprinkle with lemon and onion.

• Wrap in foil and bake in 375°F oven until salmon is thoroughly cooked, about 20 minutes. Open foil to cool. Flake fish apart with fingers to remove both skin and bones. Set fish aside; save juices.

• In steamer, cook vegetables over boiling water until tender.

• Meanwhile, in saucepan, whisk butter and flour together over medium heat until paste forms. Add milk, whisking constantly until lumps disappear. Then add dill and cooking juices, continuing to simmer until sauce thickens.

• In blender or food processor, pulse vegetables, salmon and sauce to desired consistency.

• Fill ice cube trays and freeze.

Yield: 14 to 16 cubes

SMART SARDINES

Sardines are one of the richest sources of omega-3 fatty acids. The ingredients in this recipe can be easily mashed for older babies.

I can (125 oz) sardines packed in
    tomato sauce
2 cups broccoli florets, washed
I large potato, baked, skin
    removed

OMEGA-3 AND BEHAVIOR AND LEARNING

Preliminary studies have shown a correlation between the symptoms that characterize attention deficit hyperactivity disorder (ADHD) and blood levels of omega-3 fatty acids. Boys with lower levels of omega-3 fatty acids showed more problems with behavior and learning than those with higher levels of omega-3 fatty acids.

• In steamer, cook broccoli over boiling water until tender.
• In blender or food processor, pulse sardines, potato and broccoli to achieve desired consistency.
• Fill ice cube trays and freeze.

Yield: 14 to 16 cubes

Beans and Grains

Beans and lentils are a good source of both iron and protein. By 8 or 9 months, your baby may be ready for lumpier textures, so, instead of puréeing the beans, try mashing with a fork to preserve texture. Always rinse and drain canned beans and vegetables to remove excess salt.

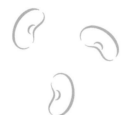

TUSCAN TOMATO AND CHICKPEAS

1/2 onion, diced

1 tbsp olive oil

2 zucchini, washed, trimmed and
   diced

1 can (14 oz) chopped tomatoes

1 can (19 oz) chickpeas, rinsed and
   drained

Pinch cumin (optional)

1/3 cup chopped fresh basil
   (optional)

• In frying pan, heat oil over low heat; sauté onion until translucent, about 5 minutes. Add zucchini and continue to sauté, stirring occasionally, for 20 minutes.

• Add tomatoes, chickpeas and cumin (if using) and simmer, partially covered, for 30 minutes. Stir occasionally.

• Remove from heat, add basil (if using) and stir. Mash with fork.

• Fill ice cube trays and freeze.

Yield: 16 cubes

IS IT SAFE TO FEED BABY A VEGETARIAN DIET?

In adults, the health benefits of reducing animal fat intake are well known; however, whether vegetarian diets are healthy for a growing baby remains controversial. It is possible to develop serious vitamin, mineral and fatty acid deficiencies, as the requirement for these nutrients is higher in babies and children than it is in adults. It is known, for example, that the risk of iron deficiency is much higher for those on a vegetarian diet. A strict vegan diet (without dairy or animal products) is not safe for children under 2. Vegetarian parents may benefit from a consultation from a pediatric dietitian to ensure baby's nutrient demands are being met.

NAVY BEANS

1 tbsp olive oil

1/2 onion, diced

1 zucchini, washed, trimmed and
diced

1 sweet red pepper, washed,
peeled with potato peeler and
diced

1 can (14 oz) chopped tomatoes

1 carrot, washed, peeled and
diced

1 can (19 oz) navy beans, rinsed
and drained

1/2 cup chopped fresh basil
(optional)

• In frying pan, heat oil over medium heat; sauté onion until translucent, about 5 minutes. Add zucchini and red pepper; continue to sauté for another 15 minutes, stirring occasionally.

• Add tomatoes, carrot and beans to frying pan; simmer, partially covered, for another 30 minutes.

• Remove from heat, add basil (if using) and stir. Mash with fork.

• Fill ice cube trays and freeze.

Yield: 16 cubes

GREEN LENTILS

1 tbsp olive oil

1/2 onion, diced

1 stalk celery, washed, trimmed
and sliced

1 clove garlic, crushed (optional)

1 tsp curry powder

1 can (14 oz) diced tomatoes

1 can (19 oz) green lentils, drained
and rinsed

3 tbsp tomato paste

1/4 cup chopped fresh cilantro or
basil (optional)

• In frying pan, heat oil over medium heat; sauté onion and celery until onion is translucent, about 5 minutes. Reduce heat; stir in garlic and curry powder. Continue to sauté for another 5 minutes.

• Add tomatoes, lentils and tomato paste; sauté for another 35 minutes.

• Remove from heat and add cilantro or basil (if using). Mix thoroughly. Mash with fork.

• Fill ice cube trays and freeze.

Yield: 16 cubes

THE IMPORTANCE OF ZINC

Dietary zinc plays diverse roles in metabolic functions of the body. Growth velocity, immune function, appetite, cognitive function and behavior are all dependent on sufficient zinc levels in the diet. Some diaper rashes may suggest zinc deficiency and will improve by increasing dietary zinc and by applying a diaper cream containing zinc. Adequate levels of zinc are also thought to help protect the body from metal toxicity such as lead poisoning. The best supply of zinc is from animal sources such as meat, eggs and human milk. Zinc is also available in legumes, potatoes and whole grains but is not as well absorbed as animal sources of zinc. Fortified breakfast cereals and baby cereals are also good sources for infants and children.

NOTE: Couscous is a wheat product and therefore should not be served to babies with wheat allergy or gluten intolerance.

SWEET PEPPER COUSCOUS

1/2 onion, diced

1 tbsp plus 1 tsp olive oil

1 sweet red pepper, washed, peeled with potato peeler and finely diced

1 sweet yellow pepper, washed, peeled and finely diced

1/4 cup chopped fresh basil (optional)

1/2 cup water

1/2 cup couscous

• In frying pan, heat 1 tbsp oil over medium heat; sauté onion until translucent, about 5 minutes. Add peppers and continue to sauté for 25 minutes. Stir in basil (if using) and set aside.

• In saucepan, add 1 tsp olive oil to water and bring to a boil.

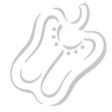

LIZ'S COUSCOUS

1/2 cup diced onion

1 tbsp plus 1 tsp olive oil

2 zucchinis, washed, trimmed and
finely diced

1/2 cup water

1/2 cup couscous

• In frying pan, heat 1 tbsp oil over medium heat; sauté onion until translucent, about 5 minutes. Add zucchini and continue to sauté until zucchini is thoroughly cooked, about 25 minutes.

• In saucepan, add 1 tsp olive oil to water and bring to a boil. Pour couscous into water, cover with lid and remove from heat. Allow to stand for 5 minutes. Fluff with fork and allow to stand for another 5 minutes. Once couscous is fluffy in consistency, add zucchini and mix thoroughly.

• *Tip:* For younger babies, you may choose to use a blender or food processor to purée couscous before freezing.

• Fill ice cube trays and freeze.

Yield: 10 cubes

• Pour couscous into water, cover with lid and remove from heat. Allow to stand for 5 minutes. Fluff with fork and allow to stand for another 5 minutes. Once couscous is fluffy in consistency, add peppers and mix thoroughly.

• *Tip:* For younger babies you may choose to use a blender or food processor to purée couscous before freezing.

• Fill ice cube trays and freeze.

Yield: 10 cubes

VEGETABLE BARLEY RISOTTO

This tempting and nutrient-packed dish makes a hearty accompaniment to a family meal. Just add salt and pepper to taste. Barley should not be consumed by babies diagnosed with gluten intolerance.

I cup barley

2 tbsp olive oil

I/2 onion, diced

I stalk celery, washed, trimmed
    and finely diced

I carrot, washed, peeled and grated
    using a cheese grater

I/2 bulb fennel, outer layer
    removed, sections separated
    and washed, finely diced

I clove garlic, mashed (optional)

3 I/2 cups Salt-Free Chicken
    Stock (recipe, page 76)

I tbsp chopped fresh parsley
    (optional)

- Rinse barley and set aside.
- In frying pan, heat oil over medium heat; sauté vegetables and garlic (if using) until vegetables are tender, about 10 minutes.
- Add barley and continue to stir. Add enough stock to cover barley; bring to a boil. Reduce heat and simmer, stirring occasionally, for 30 to 35 minutes. Add stock as needed to keep the barley covered. Once cooked, barley should be tender but firm.
- Add parsley (if using); stir.
- *Tip:* For younger babies you may choose to use a blender or food processor to purée barley before freezing.
- Fill ice cube trays and freeze.

Yield: 16 cubes

QUINOA RISOTTO

Although considered a whole grain, quinoa is actually a seed. It is an excellent source of protein and also contains iron, vitamin E, zinc, potassium and riboflavin.

1/2 cup quinoa

I tbsp olive oil

I 1/2 cups Salt-Free Chicken Stock
   (recipe, page 76)

1/3 cup frozen peas

I handful of spinach, washed,
   tough stems removed, and
   chopped

I tomato, washed, seeded and
   finely diced

• In saucepan, sauté quinoa in oil over medium heat for 3 to 4 minutes. Add stock and bring to a boil. Reduce heat to low, cover and simmer for 20 minutes.
• Stir in peas, spinach and tomatoes and cook for another 5 minutes. When done, quinoa will be translucent.
• Remove from heat and stir.
• Fill ice cube trays and freeze.

Yield: 12 cubes

HERBAL MEDICATIONS, REMEDIES AND TEAS

The use of herbal products is widespread and increasing in many countries. Parents should consider potential hazards, however—especially for babies, who are more prone to toxicity than adults. Some products may not be subject to stringent manufacturing codes. This can lead to poor standardization; contamination with pesticides, heavy metals and other carcinogenic compounds; adulteration with other pharmaceuticals; and incorrect dosage and labeling. Furthermore, the claims made about some products may be unfounded. There have been many cases of serious electrolyte disturbances and other toxic effects in babies and children given these products. The bottom line: herbal preparations are not recommended for babies.

Soy

Soybeans, also called edamame, are used to make a variety of products, including tofu and soy milk. Soy is an excellent source of protein and contains omega-3 essential fatty acids. Soy is also a source of vitamins and minerals, most notably calcium, iron and folate. However, soy protein is also a common source of food allergies. If your infant has shown any signs of atopic disease (allergies, asthma and eczema) and/or is considered high risk for developing allergies, talk to your doctor or health care professional before introducing soy.

EDAMAME PURÉE

I cup frozen soybeans
1/2 cup water

• In saucepan, bring soybeans and water to a boil. Cover, reduce heat and simmer for 3 to 4 minutes, or until beans are tender.
• With handheld immersion blender, purée beans and water until smooth. Allow to cool.
• Pour into ice cube trays and freeze.

Yield: 6 to 8 cubes

MANGO TOFU MASH

Because of its creamy texture, silken tofu mixes well with any fruit or vegetable purée. You can substitute a cube of your baby's favorite purée for the mango in this recipe. You can also mix tofu with mashed fresh fruit.

I cube mango purée, defrosted
2 tbsp silken tofu

• In a small bowl, combine mango and tofu and whisk until smooth.

Yield: 1 serving

Pasta

Most babies love pasta. And the best part is, it's good for them. It is an excellent source of both B vitamins and complex carbohydrates. Complex carbohydrates provide a sustained source of energy that will last throughout the day. When choosing pasta, opt for whole grain or enriched pasta. The enrichment process replaces some of the vitamins and minerals that were lost when the flour was refined. Some imported Italian pastas are not made with enriched flour. To find out if the pasta you are buying is enriched, look for the following nutrients on the ingredients list: iron, folic acid, riboflavin, niacin and thiamin.

Tiny pastines, traditionally used in soups, do not need to be puréed. Larger shapes such as penne or rotini can be served as finger food. Many of the following recipes can be made in bulk, then puréed and frozen. To cook dried pasta, place it in boiling, lightly salted water. Add a dash of oil and stir immediately to prevent pasta from sticking. For younger babies, cook 1 minute longer than recommended on the package. Once cooked, drain and rinse pasta under cool water. This rinses off both salt and starch, preventing the pasta from sticking.

Many of the vegetable purées make delicious pasta sauces. Just heat 2 cubes of your baby's favorite purée and mix with 1 oz of cooked pasta and 1 tbsp of grated cheese (after 9 months).

Pasta is a wheat product and should not be eaten by babies diagnosed with wheat allergy or gluten intolerance. Please note, however, that gluten- and wheat-free pastas are now readily available at most grocery stores and these pastas can be substituted in the following recipes.

MINESTRONE

I tbsp olive oil

1/4 onion, diced

I zucchini, washed, trimmed and
   sliced

I can (14 oz) chopped tomatoes

2 cups Salt-Free Chicken Stock
   (recipe, page 76)

I 1/2 cups broccoli florets, washed

2 carrots, washed, peeled and
   sliced

1/2 cup canned chickpeas, drained
   and rinsed

1/2 cup macaroni

I handful spinach, washed and
   tough stems removed

1/4 cup chopped fresh basil
   (optional)

• In large pot, heat oil over medium heat; sauté onion until translucent, about 5 minutes. Add both zucchini and tomatoes; sauté for another 20 minutes. Stir occasionally.

• Add chicken stock, broccoli, carrots, chickpeas and pasta; bring to a boil. Reduce heat and simmer, partially covered, for 20 minutes.

• Add spinach and basil (if using); continue to simmer for another 10 minutes. The consistency should be that of a thick stew. If there is too much liquid, remove lid for last 5 to 10 minutes of cooking.

• With a slotted spoon, place vegetables, pasta and chickpeas in blender or food processor. Set leftover cooking juices aside.

• Purée, adding leftover juices as needed to achieve desired consistency.

• Pour into ice cube trays and freeze.

Yield: 18 to 20 cubes

CHICKEN NOODLE STEW

I chicken breast, cut in cubes

I sprig fresh tarragon (optional)

2 cups water

I/3 cup macaroni

I stalk celery, washed, trimmed
and sliced

2 carrots, washed, peeled and
sliced

I/4 onion, cut in half

I potato, washed, peeled and cut
in cubes

I/4 cup chopped fresh parsley
(optional)

• In large pot, place chicken and tarragon (if using) in water and bring to a boil.

• Add pasta, celery, carrots, onion and potato; reduce heat and simmer, partially covered, until vegetables are tender, about 25 minutes. Stir occasionally. The consistency should be that of a thick stew. If there is too much liquid, remove lid for last 5 to 10 minutes of cooking.

• Remove from heat. Add parsley (if using) and stir.

• Using a slotted spoon, place vegetables, pasta and chicken in blender or food processor. Set leftover cooking juices aside.

• Purée, adding juices as needed to achieve desired consistency.

• Pour into ice cube trays and freeze.

Yield: 18 to 20 cubes

FOOD REFUSAL

Beginning at about 8 months it is common for babies to refuse meals. They demonstrate this by shutting the mouth, turning the head or throwing food. Often the refusal occurs even if the baby is hungry and before the meal is even tasted. It is very important that parents recognize that this is a normal developmental stage and it does not represent defiance. It may also signal a desire for independence and the opportunity for baby to feed herself. Giving baby a spoon to hold and encouraging self-feeding attempts may help.

Nevertheless, refusal often persists and can become very frustrating for parents. Resist force-feeding or punishing your baby. Instead increase nutritious snacks to alleviate hunger. This does not set a bad precedent; at this young age, a baby does not understand that refusing at one time leads to snacks at another. Continue to include your baby in family mealtimes but postpone the essential "three square meals" until later in childhood. If your baby has persistent low appetite, discuss the possibility of iron deficiency with your physician.

WHAT ARE NURSING CARIES?

Nursing caries or "nursing bottle syndrome" refers to the damaging effects of continuous bottle-feeding to the teeth. If teeth are continuously bathed in nutrient-containing liquids such as milk, fruit juice or other sugar-containing drinks there is a continual supply of sugar on which dental bacteria proliferate and this may cause cavities. This is most likely to occur in a baby over 12 months old who is given a bottle for sleep or as a pacifier. When the baby falls asleep liquid may pool in the mouth and coat the teeth. A baby who discards the bottle prior to falling asleep is at much less risk than one who falls asleep with the bottle in her mouth. Beware of propping up the bottle so baby can self-feed, which can contribute to dental caries and cause choking. Liquids other than breast milk should be given in a cup by 12 months of age, and try to switch to water at bedtime if a bottle is necessary to fall asleep.

Tooth brushing should begin with the appearance of the first tooth and occur twice a day, using a baby toothbrush with a smear of toothpaste.

VEGETABLE PRIMAVERA

This recipe can also be served with cheese (after age 9 months). Defrost 3 cubes and mix in a saucepan over low heat with 1 tbsp of grated cheddar cheese.

1 tbsp olive oil

1/4 onion, diced

1 zucchini, washed, trimmed and
   sliced

1 sweet red pepper, washed,
   peeled with potato peeler and
   diced

1 yellow pepper, washed, peeled
   and diced

1 can (14 oz) tomatoes, packed in
   their own juice

1 1/2 cups broccoli florets, washed

1/4 cup water

1/3 cup chopped fresh basil
   (optional)

1 cup (8 oz) dried pasta, cooked

• In frying pan, heat oil over medium heat; sauté onion until translucent, about 5 minutes. Add zucchini and peppers; continue to sauté, stirring occasionally, for 20 minutes.

• Stir in tomatoes, broccoli and water; simmer, partially covered, until broccoli is tender, about 20 minutes.

• Remove from heat; stir in basil (if using) and cooked pasta.

• In blender or food processor, purée mixture to desired consistency. Let cool.

• Pour into ice cube trays and freeze.

Yield: 22 to 24 cubes

Eggs

Eggs, with their soft, creamy texture, are seemingly the perfect food for infants. They are high in protein, contain both iron and omega-3 fatty acids and are one of the few dietary sources of vitamin D. However, egg allergy is one of the most common allergies among infants and it can be virulent.

In the past, well-cooked egg yolk was introduced at 6 months and egg whites at a year, since egg whites contain at least twenty-three different glycoproteins, which can be problematic in sensitive individuals. However, recent findings suggest there is no evidence that delaying eggs will reduce your baby's risk of developing an allergy to eggs. If your infant has shown no signs of atopic disease (allergies, asthma and eczema) and is not considered high risk for developing allergies, there seems no reason to further delay eggs. Given this, it only seems sensible to start with a well-cooked egg yolk. Assuming your baby doesn't have an adverse reaction, you may proceed with the whole egg.

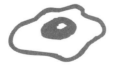

HARD-BOILED EGG YOLK

Cut into bite-size pieces, egg yolks are the perfect finger food.

I egg
I tsp breast milk or formula
   (approx)

• Place egg in saucepan and cover with water so that there is at least 1 inch of water above egg.
• Cover pot with lid and bring to a full boil over medium heat.
• Once water comes to a full boil, remove from heat and let stand for 17 minutes.
• Drain and rinse egg under cold water.
• Once cool, peel and discard shell and egg white.
• Mash egg yoke with breast milk or formula.

Yield: 1 serving

BABY'S FIRST SCRAMBLE

I egg
I tbsp breast milk or formula
I tsp canola oil (or salt-free butter
   after 9 months)

• In a small bowl, mix egg and milk together.
• Evenly spread canola oil over saucepan and place over medium-low heat.
• Pour egg into saucepan and scramble until thoroughly cooked, about 5 to 7 minutes.

Yield: 1 serving

EGG AND AVOCADO MASH

I hard-boiled egg, shell removed
I/4 of an avocado

• In a small bowl, mash egg and avocado together. Serve immediately, before avocado turns brown.

Yield: 1 serving

Finger Foods

At around 8 months of age your baby may express an interest in feeding herself: this is the time to introduce finger foods. When introducing finger foods for the first time choose soft fruits (bananas, peaches or pears) or steamed vegetables. Teething babies may enjoy eating Melba toast, dry bread crusts, or bagels. Starting a meal with finger foods is often a good way to distract baby while the main course is being prepared.

Your baby should eat finger foods only when sitting upright and supervised by an adult. Some foods are considered risky because they can cause choking and therefore should be avoided by both babies and toddlers. See Proceed with Caution (page 62). Remember when serving fruit to peel and remove either the seeds or the pit.

At around 1 year of age it is not unusual for your baby to refuse to be fed by you altogether. Often the best way to encourage your baby to eat is to offer a variety of finger foods. At this stage your baby may enjoy eating pieces of cooked meat or shredded cheese. A well-balanced meal can be made entirely of finger foods. An easy way to prepare such meals in advance is to poach a chicken breast, and steam half a bunch of broccoli and two carrots. Cut up chicken, broccoli and carrots into finger-size pieces, divide into individual portions and freeze in freezer bags. *To serve:* Defrost. Heat in oven until warm.

What follows are some ideas for a smorgasbord of finger foods.

FRUIT Peeled raw fruits such as bananas, pears, peaches, papaya or blueberries are good introductory finger foods. Seedless grapes should be cut lengthwise several times. Harder fruits such as apples can be grated or served in larger pieces that your baby can hold and chew on. (Cold apples can help soothe sore gums.) Indulge your baby's need for independence by serving a bowl of interesting fruit from which he can choose and serve himself.

VEGETABLES Steamed cauliflower, broccoli, beans or peas are tasty. Carrots should be served either soft-cooked and cut lengthwise or grated. Cherry tomatoes cut in quarters, shredded lettuce, ripe avocados and thin slices of cucumber can all be served raw. Potatoes and yams cut in wedges and roasted are a healthy alternative to french fries. Steamed vegetable sticks are often a great appetizer before you offer up the main course.

BREADS AND CEREAL You may introduce toast, whole-grain crackers and rice cakes at this stage. Cooked pasta can be served either on its own or with a thick sauce. Whole-grain cereal such as Cheerios, cornflakes or Spoon-Size Shredded Wheat can be served without milk. If your baby begins to lose interest in your purées, try serving them as a dip with either toast strips or precooked vegetable sticks.

MEATS AND PROTEINS Your baby may enjoy eating small pieces of cooked chicken, beef, fish and cubes of soft tofu. Whatever meat you are cooking for dinner, make sure there will be some left over for baby's lunch the next day. The fish sticks and chicken fingers in this book are popular. Serve them with homemade Tomato Sauce (recipe, page 124) or some of the vegetable purées. Dipping fish sticks into Florets and Cheese Sauce (recipe, page 131) is an entertaining way for your baby to eat a well-balanced meal.

DAIRY PRODUCTS Dairy products are introduced around 9 months. Cheese can be served either grated or cut into thin slices, and most babies enjoy cheese melted on bread cut into strips.

At 6 months some babies are ready to eat 3 meals a day. If this is the case, offer more fortified infant cereal. The meal planners are guidelines only and should not take precedent over your baby's cues for hunger and satiety.

WEEK 1

Breakfast	Breast or Bottle, Single-Grain Baby Cereal (Rice)
Mid-A.M. Snack	Breast or Bottle
Lunch	Breast or Bottle
Mid-P.M. Snack	Breast or Bottle
Dinner	Breast or Bottle Single-Grain Baby Cereal (Rice) (if desired)
Before Bed	Breast or Bottle

WEEK 2

Breakfast	Breast or Bottle, Single-Grain Baby Cereal (Rice)
Mid-A.M. Snack	Breast or Bottle
Lunch	Breast or Bottle
Mid-P.M. Snack	Breast or Bottle
Dinner	Baby's First Chicken Purée
Before Bed	Breast or Bottle

WEEK 3

Breakfast	Breast or Bottle, Single-Grain Baby Cereal (Barley)
Mid-A.M. Snack	Breast or Bottle
Lunch	Breast or Bottle, Mashed Avocado or Butternut Squash
Mid-P.M. Snack	Breast or Bottle
Dinner	Baby's First Beef Purée
Before Bed	Breast or Bottle

WEEK 4

Breakfast	Breast or Bottle, Fruit Cereal
Mid-A.M. Snack	Breast or Bottle
Lunch	Breast or Bottle, Baby's First Fish
Mid-P.M. Snack	Breast or Bottle
Dinner	Chicken and Yams
Before Bed	Breast or Bottle

Baby may also wake for additional feeds during the night.
You may mix any of the purées with baby cereal for palatability and increased iron.

FROM SIX TO NINE MONTHS

SAMPLE DAILY MEAL PLANNER: FROM 7 TO 8 MONTHS OF AGE

DAY 1

Breakfast	Breast or Bottle, Single-Grain Baby Cereal (Rice)
Mid-A.M. Snack	Breast or Bottle
Lunch	Mashed Banana, Whole Wheat Toast Strips
Mid-P.M. Snack	Breast or Bottle
Dinner	Baby's First Chicken Purée
Before Bed	Breast or Bottle

DAY 2

Breakfast	Breast or Bottle, Single-Grain Baby Cereal (Oats or Barley)
Mid-A.M. Snack	Breast or Bottle
Lunch	Watermelon Cereal
Mid-P.M. Snack	Breast or Bottle
Dinner	Chicken Apple Delight
Before Bed	Breast or Bottle

DAY 3

Breakfast	Breast or Bottle, Florida Breakfast
Mid-A.M. Snack	Breast or Bottle
Lunch	Vegetable Rice
Mid-P.M. Snack	Breast or Bottle
Dinner	Baby Chicken
Before Bed	Breast or Bottle

DAY 4

Breakfast	Breast or Bottle, Fruit Cereal
Mid-A.M. Snack	Breast or Bottle
Lunch	Kale and Apple Purée
Mid-P.M. Snack	Breast or Bottle
Dinner	Fish and Pear Purée
Before Bed	Breast or Bottle

SAMPLE DAILY MEAL PLANNER: FROM 7 TO 8 MONTHS OF AGE

DAY 5

Breakfast	**Breast or Bottle, Single-Grain Baby Cereal (Oats or Barley)**
Mid-A.M. Snack	**Breast or Bottle**
Lunch	**Watermelon Cereal**
Mid-P.M. Snack	**Breast or Bottle**
Dinner	**Chicken Apple Delight**
Before Bed	**Breast or Bottle**

DAY 7

Breakfast	**Breast or Bottle, Baby Cereal (Mixed Grain)**
Mid-A.M. Snack	**Breast or Bottle**
Lunch	**Fruit Trio**
Mid-P.M. Snack	**Breast or Bottle**
Dinner	**Easy Beef Hash**
Before Bed	**Breast or Bottle**

Baby may also wake for additional feeds during the night.

You may mix any of the purées with baby cereal for palatability and increased iron.

DAY 6

Breakfast	**Breast or Bottle, Single-Grain Baby Cereal (Oats) and Pear Purée**
Mid-A.M. Snack	**Breast or Bottle**
Lunch	**Vegetable Rice**
Mid-P.M. Snack	**Breast or Bottle**
Dinner	**Chicken and Winter Vegetables**
Before Bed	**Breast or Bottle**

DAY 1

Breakfast	Breast or Bottle, Watermelon Cereal
Mid-A.M. Snack	Breast or Bottle, Okanagan Summer Salad
Lunch	Pork and Apple Purée
Mid-P.M. Snack	Breast or Bottle
Dinner	Vichyssoise, Mashed Banana
Before Bed	Breast or Bottle

DAY 2

Breakfast	Breast or Bottle, Single-Grain Cereal (Oats), Mashed Banana
Mid-A.M. Snack	Breast or Bottle, Mashed Avocado
Lunch	Chicken Apple Delight
Mid-P.M. Snack	Breast or Bottle
Dinner	Vegetable Stew
Before Bed	Breast or Bottle

DAY 3

Breakfast	Breast or Bottle, Single-Grain Baby Cereal (Oats), Apple Purée
Mid-A.M. Snack	Breast or Bottle, Vegetable Trio
Lunch	Chicken Noodle Stew, Mashed Pear
Mid-P.M. Snack	Breast or Bottle
Dinner	Mashed Avocado, Mashed Banana
Before Bed	Breast or Bottle

DAY 4

Breakfast	Breast or Bottle, Single-Grain Baby Cereal (Rice) Mashed Banana
Mid-A.M. Snack	Breast or Bottle, Cucumber
Lunch	Ratatouille, Mashed Avocado
Mid-P.M. Snack	Breast or Bottle
Dinner	West Coast Salmon, Pear Purée
Before Bed	Breast or Bottle

DAY 5

Breakfast	**Breast or Bottle, Baby Cereal (Mixed-Grain), Mashed Banana**
Mid-A.M. Snack	**Breast or Bottle, Edamame Purée**
Lunch	**Thanksgiving Dinner**
Mid-P.M. Snack	**Breast or Bottle**
Dinner	**Vegetable Primavera, Melon**
Before Bed	**Breast or Bottle**

DAY 6

Breakfast	**Breast or Bottle, Single-Grain Baby Cereal (Oats)**
Mid-A.M. Snack	**Breast or Bottle, Spaghetti Squash Smash**
Lunch	**Hard-Boiled Egg Yolk, Whole Wheat Toast Strips**
Mid-P.M. Snack	**Breast or Bottle**
Dinner	**Maxwell's Minted Lamb**
Before Bed	**Breast or Bottle**

DAY 7

Breakfast	**Breast or Bottle, Baby Cereal (Mixed Grain)**
Mid-A.M. Snack	**Breast or Bottle, Broccoli and Sweet Potato Purée**
Lunch	**Tuscan Tomato and Chickpeas**
Mid-P.M. Snack	**Breast or Bottle**
Dinner	**Red Snapper Salsa Provencal**
Before Bed	**Breast or Bottle**

Baby may also wake for additional feeds during the night.

You may mix any of the purées with baby cereal for palatability and increased iron.

FROM SIX TO NINE MONTHS

119

From Nine to Twelve Months

By 9 months of age your baby will enjoy eating slightly lumpier textures. Instead of puréeing the food, try mashing it with a fork or chopping it into baby-bite-size pieces. Cut down on the puréeing time to provide lumpier and more interesting textures. Although your baby is not likely to become proficient with a spoon until at least 12 months, he should be encouraged in his attempts to self-feed. With each little triumph his confidence will grow. At this stage some babies may reject being spoon-fed altogether, while others continue for many months. Fortunately, healthy meals can be made up entirely of finger foods (see Finger Foods, page 113).

At this stage baby appetites and sizes vary greatly. Provided your little one is developing normally, you need not be overly concerned about comparing him with other babies. Offer nutritious snacks and meals and be reassured that no healthy baby will starve himself. There is little correlation between big babies and overweight adults. Please vary serving sizes according to your baby's appetite.

This is a sensible time to introduce calcium-rich dairy products, such as yogurt and cheese. Introducing them much earlier may increase the risk of gastrointestinal bleeding. Cow's milk for drinking should be postponed until 12 months.

Children under the age of 2 should be served full-fat dairy products. Avoid soy, rice and other vegetarian beverages until 2 years as the fat content, equivalent to 2% milk, is too low for babies.

Babies tend to love cheese and yogurt. All cheeses must be pasteurized. Cheddar, mozzarella, Edam, Gouda and cottage cheese tend to be popular with babies. To avoid the additives found in many commercial yogurts, choose a plain high-fat yogurt (any yogurt above 3% milk fat) and mix it with your baby's favorite fruit or vegetable purée.

These recommendations may differ if your baby has shown signs of atopic disease (allergies, eczema or asthma) or if you have allergies in the family. If this is the case, consult your doctor before adding dairy products to your infant's diet.

The recipes in this section are more complex; some contain foods from all four food groups. Many of the recipes contain dairy products and most can be made in bulk and should be puréed, mashed or finely chopped until desired consistency is reached.

CHARLIE'S CHEESY CHICKEN

Charlie's Cheesy Chicken combines very well with a variety of vegetable purées. Defrost 2 cubes Cheesy Chicken and 2 cubes broccoli purée. Combine in saucepan over low heat, and serve. Try a variety of other delicious combinations by substituting any of the vegetable purées for the broccoli.

1 recipe Poached Chicken Breast
    (page 36)
1/2 cup cottage cheese
1/3 cup (1.5 oz) grated cheddar
    cheese
1/4 cup Salt-Free Chicken Stock
(2 to 3 cubes) (recipe, page 76)
or
leftover poaching water

• In blender or food processor, purée chicken, cottage cheese and cheddar cheese. Add stock, as needed, to achieve desired consistency.
• Pour into ice cube trays and freeze.

Yield: 14 cubes

FIT FOR LIFE

Life expectancy in many nations consistently exceeds predicted forecasts. In the 1920s life expectancy averaged age 65. In 1990 it was 85. Now it is believed that a baby girl born in Japan or France (countries with the highest life expectancy) has a 50-percent chance of living to 100! With the prospect of this longevity, it is important to equip children with strong skeletons. Osteoporosis is a disease that causes a stooped spine and weak, easily broken bones. Symptoms usually begin after age 50 but prevention begins in infancy with the development of strong bones from adequate calcium intake. Plenty of calcium, exercise and vitamin D will help to reduce the risk of osteoporosis. Dairy is the best source of calcium, but adequate intake may be achieved with alternative sources. Other sources of calcium include tofu, white beans, navy beans, sardines, canned salmon with bones, instant oats and leafy greens. Most infant cereals also contain skim milk powder.

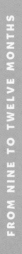

TOMATO SAUCE

Many of the following recipes will require a cube of tomato sauce. This simple recipe can form the basis of a delicious pasta sauce for the whole family. Just add garlic, salt and pepper to taste.

1/2 onion, finely diced

1 tbsp olive oil

1 can (14 oz) diced tomatoes

2 tbsp tomato paste

1/4 cup water

1/3 cup chopped fresh basil

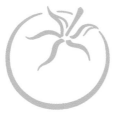

SKINNED SEEDED TOMATOES

Some of the recipes in this book will require tomatoes that have been skinned and seeded. To prepare, plunge tomatoes in a saucepan of boiling water for 30 seconds. Remove from water with slotted spoon; allow to cool. Slit skin with a knife and peel. Cut tomato into quarters; remove seeds.

• In frying pan, heat olive oil over low heat; sauté onion until translucent.

• Add tomatoes, tomato paste and water; bring to a boil.

• Turn down heat and add basil; simmer, partially covered, for 30 minutes, stirring occasionally.

• Pour into ice cube trays and freeze.

Yield: 10 cubes

TOMATO AND CHEESE PASTA

As your baby begins to declare her independence, pasta and sauce is a good choice. Although messy, individual pieces can be grasped by little hands.

1/4 cup (2 oz) dried pasta
2 cubes Tomato Sauce (recipe,
    page 124)
I tbsp grated mozzarella cheese

• Defrost cubes of tomato sauce.
• In saucepan, cook pasta in boiling water. Drain pasta and rinse under cool water.
• In separate saucepan, combine tomato sauce, pasta and mozzarella cheese over low heat. Stir until cheese melts.
• Using blender or food processor, pulse to desired consistency.

Yield: 1 serving

CHICKEN CACCIATORE

2 cubes Charlie's Cheesy Chicken
    (recipe, page 123)
I cube Tomato Sauce (recipe,
    page 124)

• Defrost cubes. Heat in saucepan over low heat until warm. Serve.

Yield: 1 serving

125

BROCCOLI SURPRISE

Tomato sauce mixes very well with most vegetables. To make other delicious combinations, follow this recipe substituting your baby's favorite purée for the broccoli.

I cube Tomato Sauce (recipe, page 124)
2 cubes broccoli purée (recipe, page 153)
I tbsp grated cheddar cheese

• Defrost cubes.
• In saucepan, mix over low heat. Add cheese, stirring occasionally.
• Remove from heat; cool to room temperature.

Yield: 1 serving

HOW TALL WILL BABY GROW?

Since height is partly genetically determined, it is possible to estimate a child's adult height based on the parents' height. The estimate has a range of +/- 18 cm (3.15 inches).

FOR A BOY

$$\frac{\text{(Father's height in cm + Mother's height in cm + 13)}}{2}$$

FOR A GIRL

$$\frac{\text{(Father's height in cm - 13 + Mother's height in cm)}}{2}$$

SOLE WITH SALSA AND CHEESE

8 oz sole fillet

2 tomatoes, skinned, seeded and diced (see Skinned Seeded Tomatoes, page 124)

I tbsp finely diced onion

I tbsp chopped fresh parsley (optional)

1/2 cup (2 oz) grated cheddar cheese

- Place fish on tinfoil.
- In bowl, mix tomatoes, onion and parsley (if using). Coat fish with this tomato salsa and wrap in foil. Bake in 375°F oven until fish is thoroughly cooked, about 20 minutes.
- Open foil to allow cooling. Flake fish apart with fingers to remove bones.
- In blender or food processor, pulse fish, tomato salsa and cheese to achieve desired consistency.
- Fill ice cube trays and freeze.

Yield: 10 to 12 cubes

LASAGNA MASH

I can (14 oz) diced tomatoes

1/4 cup water

8 cubes stewing beef

1/4 onion, diced

I carrot, washed, peeled and sliced

1/2 cup (4 oz) macaroni or other dried pasta

I tbsp chopped fresh basil (optional)

1/3 cup (1.5 oz) grated mozzarella cheese

1/2 cup cottage cheese

- In saucepan, combine tomatoes, water, beef, onion, carrot and pasta; bring to a boil. Reduce heat and simmer, partially covered, stirring occasionally, until meat is thoroughly cooked, 25 to 30 minutes. The consistency should be that of a thick stew. If you feel there is too much liquid, remove the lid for the last 5 to 10 minutes of cooking.
- Remove from heat; add basil (if using) and cheeses. Stir until cheese melts.
- In blender or food processor, pulse mixture to desired consistency.
- Fill ice cube trays and freeze.

Yield: 16 to 18 cubes

PESTICIDES AND HORMONES IN PRODUCE AND MEAT

Controversy regarding hormone and pesticide use has caused many people to "go organic." Is this extra expense necessary? Organic food is produced according to legally regulated standards. Produce is grown without the use of synthetic pesticides, fertilizers and herbicides, and animals are reared without the use of antibiotics and hormones. In Canada hormones are routinely given to beef cattle to speed up their growth, ensuring they gain less fat and more muscle. In Canada hormones are not given to dairy cattle, chicken, pigs or sheep. Although Health Canada states that meat from animals treated with homones does not pose a threat to human health, some scientists remain concerned. They fear trace residue of hormones in meat could disrupt hormonal balances in the body. Given these concerns, you may want to consider buying organic beef if feasible.

Pesticides are strictly researched and monitored by regulatory bodies. Only those pesticides known not to cause adverse effects at reasonable levels of consumption are approved. Parents should not restrict produce consumption because of pesticide fears as there is overwhelming scientific consensus that the health benefits of eating produce far outweigh any possible pesticide risks. To minimize risk, choose produce free of dirt, cuts, insect holes or mold, wash produce thoroughly in water and remove outer skin or leaves. There is little evidence that "organically grown" foods are safer or more nutritious than foods conventionally grown. In fact, many organic growers use "environmental" pesticides such as sulfur, nicotine and copper, and although thought to be less toxic the relative risk remains unclear. While organic farming practices are better for the environment, the decision to go organic is a personal choice. Regardless of what you decide, what is most important is that your baby is eating a wide variety of fruit and vegetables.

SPINACH AND CHEESE

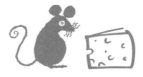

I potato, washed, peeled and cut
  in cubes
4 handfuls of spinach, washed and
  tough stems removed
1/3 cup (1.5 oz) grated cheddar
  cheese, loosely packed
1/2 cup cottage cheese
1/4 cup Vegetable Stock (2 to 3
  cubes) (recipe, page 58)
or
leftover cooking water (optional)

• In saucepan of boiling water, cook potato for 20 minutes; drain, reserving leftover cooking water.
• In steamer, cook spinach for 5 minutes.
• In blender or food processor, purée vegetables and cheese. If mixture seems too thick, add either stock or leftover cooking water as required.
• Pour into ice cube trays and freeze.

Yield: 10 to 12 cubes

WHAT ABOUT SALT?

Sodium is an essential dietary nutrient that plays an important role in metabolism and maintenance of blood pressure. Sodium occurs naturally in many foods, including cow's milk, human milk, cheese, vegetables and grains. It also can be added to foods in the form of salt. In adults, an excess of sodium can raise blood pressure and cause significant health problems in later life. As it is not clear what the consequences of excess sodium are for infants, it seems wise not to use added salt when preparing baby food. For older children, moderate use of salt in a few selected foods is acceptable. Most important, parents should consider their habits and model moderate intake so that as the child begins to eat from the family table, he learns not to over-salt.

SOLE, VEGETABLES AND CHEESE

10 oz sole fillet or any white fish

Dash lemon juice

1 tbsp finely diced onion

2 cups broccoli florets, washed

2 carrots, washed, peeled and
    sliced

1 tsp of flour (approx)

1 tsp butter (approx)

1/2 cup breast milk or formula
    (3.25% milk after age 12
    months)

1/2 cup (2 oz) grated cheddar
    cheese

• Place fish on tinfoil. Sprinkle with lemon juice and onion. Wrap fish in foil. Bake in 375°F oven until fish is thoroughly cooked, about 20 minutes.

• Open foil to allow cooling. Flake fish apart with fingers to remove bones. Set fish aside; reserve cooking juices.

• Meanwhile, in steamer, cook vegetables over boiling water until tender; set aside.

• In saucepan, whisk flour and butter together over medium heat until paste forms. Add 1/4 cup milk, whisking constantly until lumps disappear. Add cheese and remainder of milk, whisking until cheese melts.

• Add cooking juices to pan; whisk until sauce thickens.

• In blender or food processor, purée vegetables, sauce and fish to desired consistency.

• Fill ice cube trays and freeze.

Yield: 14 cubes

WHY BOTHER?

Often a well-meaning parent can become discouraged by a baby's continual refusal of food. This is especially true for those who have committed to homemade baby food, investing precious time and energy in preparing nutritious meals, only to be met with refusal and protest. One may ask, why bother? Considering your child will depend on you for proper nutrition and the potential to shape food choices and consequently her health, it is important to persevere. Children who observe your commitment to nutritious eating, even if it requires more time and energy, will likely carry this philosophy with them into adulthood.

FLORETS AND CHEESE SAUCE

For older babies, steam florets and serve sauce on the side, as they will enjoy dipping veggies into the sauce. Try serving the sauce with different vegetables, such as thinly sliced steamed beans, soft-cooked carrots or quartered cherry tomatoes.

I tbsp butter

I tbsp flour (approx)

I cup breast milk or formula

I 1/2 cups (6 oz) grated, mature
   cheddar cheese, firmly packed

2 cups broccoli florets, washed

2 cups cauliflower florets, washed

• *To prepare cheese sauce:* In saucepan, whisk butter and flour together over medium heat until paste forms. Slowly add 1/2 cup of milk, whisking until lumps disappear. Continue to whisk, while adding cheese and the remaining milk. Stir until cheese melts and sauce thickens to a smooth, creamy texture.

• In steamer, cook florets over boiling water for 10 minutes. In blender or food processor, combine with cheese sauce and purée to achieve desired consistency.

• Pour into ice cube trays and freeze.

Yield: 16 cubes

QUICK CARROT AND PARSNIP AU GRATIN

3 carrots, washed, peeled and
  sliced
3 parsnips, washed, peeled and
  sliced
I cup (4 oz) grated Gruyère
  cheese
1/4 cup Vegetable Stock (2 to 3
  cubes) (recipe, page 58)
or
leftover cooking water (optional)

• In steamer, steam vegetables for 15 minutes.
• In blender or food processor, purée vegetables and cheese. If purée seems too thick, add either stock or leftover cooking water to achieve desired consistency.
• Pour into ice cube trays and freeze.

Yield: 12 to 14 cubes

BAJA CHICKEN SALAD

2 oz Poached Chicken Breast
  (recipe, page 36)
I slice avocado, washed, skin
  removed
I tbsp grated cheddar cheese
I tsp chopped fresh cilantro
  (optional)

• In blender or food processor, pulse chicken, avocado, cheese and cilantro (if using) to achieve desired consistency.

Yield: 1 serving

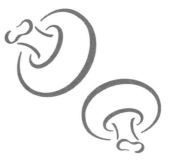

BAKED TOMATO AND ZUCCHINI AU GRATIN

This dish makes a quick and satisfying vegetable accompaniment to family meals. Just add salt and pepper to taste.

2 tbsp olive oil

4 baby zucchinis, washed, trimmed and sliced

10 mushrooms, washed and sliced

4 tomatoes, skinned and seeded, diced (see Skinned Seeded Tomatoes, page 124)

1 1/2 cups (6 oz) grated cheddar cheese

1/4 cup (1 oz) grated Parmesan cheese

2 tbsp chopped fresh basil (optional)

• In large frying pan, heat oil over medium heat; sauté zucchini and mushrooms, stirring occasionally, until zucchini is golden brown, 25 to 30 minutes.

• In ovenproof dish, layer zucchini mixture, tomatoes and cheddar cheese. Sprinkle with Parmesan cheese and basil (if using).

• Bake in 375°F oven for 30 minutes. Remove from oven and cool.

• In blender or food processor, purée to desired consistency.

• Pour into ice cube trays and freeze.

Yield: 16 cubes

ZUCCHINI, CHICKEN AND CHEESE

I tbsp olive oil

1/4 onion, diced

I zucchini, washed, trimmed and
diced

I recipe Poached Chicken Breast
(page 36)

1/2 cup (2 oz) grated cheddar
cheese

1/3 cup chopped fresh parsley
(optional)

3 tbsp high-fat (above 3%) plain
yogurt

2 tomatoes, washed, skinned,
seeded and diced (see
Skinned Seeded Tomatoes,
page 124)

• In frying pan, heat oil over medium heat; sauté onion until translucent, about 5 minutes. Add zucchini and continue to sauté until thoroughly cooked, 20 to 25 minutes. Remove from heat and cool.

• In blender or food processor, pulse zucchini mixture with chicken, cheese, parsley (if using), yogurt and tomatoes to achieve desired consistency.

• Fill ice cube trays and freeze.

Yield: 16 cubes

OKANAGAN SUMMER CHICKEN

The intriguing combination of creamy corn and peaches makes this dish a delectable treat.

2 peaches, washed

I cob corn, husked and kernels
   removed

I recipe Poached Chicken Breast
   (page 36)

• In saucepan, plunge peaches into boiling water for 30 seconds. Remove with slotted spoon and cool. Slit skin with a knife and remove. Cut peaches into quarters, removing pit.

• In steamer, steam peaches and corn over boiling water for 5 minutes. Reserve leftover cooking water.

• In blender or food processor, purée peaches, corn and chicken to achieve desired consistency. If purée seems too thick, add either leftover cooking water or unsweetened apple juice, 1 tbsp at a time.

• Fill ice cube trays and freeze.

Yield: 12 cubes

135

SUMMER SALAD

2 oz Poached Chicken Breast
(recipe, page 36)

I slice avocado, washed, skin
removed

I slice mango, washed, skin
removed

• In blender or food processor, pulse chicken, avocado and mango to desired consistency. Serve.

Yield: 1 serving

MAKING MEALTIMES FUN FOR EVERYONE

It is never too early to set the foundation for a positive attitude toward food. The best way to do this is to make sure that mealtimes are enjoyable for everyone. Although your baby may still need to be spoon-fed, it is not too early to encourage participation. While you are feeding her, place a tiny amount of purée in a bowl and allow her to explore. Although this may mean your precious purée will end up on the floor, be smushed in tiny hands or smeared on the serving tray, your baby will be grinning from ear to ear. Most messes can be minimized. Invest in a large bib and a suitable baby bowl. Newspaper under the highchair facilitates an easy clean-up.

Once your baby begins to suck her fingers, she will learn that bringing her hand to her mouth results in tasty treats. When she is able to grasp a spoon, encourage her to hold her own during mealtime. At first the spoon will just be waved in the air or banged on the tray, but slowly she will learn to dip and suck, just as she did with her fingers. Not only will your baby enjoy these initial steps toward independence, she will be distracted and it will be easier for you to spoon-feed the main course.

If your baby rejects a new purée or even a familiar favorite, don't push the issue. However nutritious the meal may be, it is not worth a power struggle, especially one you are unlikely to win. With a smile on your face, take the purée away and try again another day. The most important thing is that the meal end on a happy note for everyone.

PASTA WITH FLORETS AND CHEESE

2 cubes Florets and Cheese
    Sauce (recipe, page 131)
1/4 cup (2 oz) dried pasta

• Defrost cubes of Florets and Cheese Sauce.
• In saucepan, cook pasta in boiling water; drain.
• In separate saucepan, combine pasta and sauce over low heat until pasta is thoroughly coated.
• In blender or food processor, pulse mixture to desired consistency.

Yield: 1 serving

SUPERBABY'S SPINACH PURÉE

4 handfuls of spinach, washed and
    tough stems removed
1 large potato, washed and baked,
    skin removed
2 tbsp breast milk or formula
    (approx)

• In steamer, steam spinach over boiling water for 5 minutes.
• In blender or food processor, purée potato and spinach, adding milk as needed to achieve desired consistency.
• Pour into ice cube trays and freeze.

Yield: 10 cubes

BABY'S VEGETABLE RISOTTO

I cup arborio rice

2 tbsp olive oil

I/2 onion, diced

I baby zucchini, washed and
  trimmed

I/2 sweet red pepper, washed,
  peeled with potato peeler

I small carrot, washed, peeled and
  trimmed

2 I/2 cups Salt-Free Chicken Stock
  (recipe, page 76)

I cup (4 oz) grated Parmesan
  cheese

• Rinse rice and set aside.

• In large frying pan, heat oil over medium heat; sauté onion for 5 minutes. Meanwhile, dice both zucchini and pepper into small-bite-size pieces; grate carrot. Add zucchini, pepper and carrot to frying pan and continue to sauté until vegetables are soft, 10 to 12 minutes.

• Add rice and 1/4 cup chicken stock; simmer over medium heat. As the rice becomes dry, add more chicken stock to keep the rice moist, and stir after each addition. Chicken stock should be added in small increments throughout the entire cooking process, 20 to 25 minutes. When rice is cooked it should be just tender.

• During the last 2 minutes of cooking time, add cheese; stir until cheese melts. (Do not be tempted to add extra chicken stock, as it will cause risotto to clump.) Cool risotto.

• Fill ice cube trays and freeze.

• *Tip:* For younger babies you may choose to use a blender or food processor to pulse risotto to desired consistency.

Yield: 16 cubes

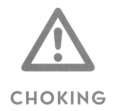

CHOKING

Each year many Canadian children die as a result of choking on food or small objects. That's why it is important to ensure all food is well puréed for babies, well mashed for older babies, or cut in small pieces for toddlers.

BABIES AND TODDLERS MUST ALWAYS BE SUPERVISED WHEN EATING.

Some foods are known to be associated with choking and should be carefully prepared, or avoided (see Proceed with Caution, page 62). Small toys, marbles, latex balloons and plastic bags can also cause choking. Parents and caregivers should be familiar with life-saving techniques and take a child safety course such as those offered by St. John Ambulance (see Appendix II, page 191).

ASSESSING THE CHOKING CHILD

1. If the child is breathing and able to make sounds or speak it is likely that natural coughing will dislodge the object. Additional maneuvers could be potentially dangerous.
2. If the child is not breathing, coughing or making sounds, back blows or chest thrusts are recommended (depending on the child's age).

TECHNIQUE IF THE CHOKING CHILD IS YOUNGER THAN I YEAR OF AGE:

1. Call an ambulance.
2. Place the infant facedown at an angle of 60 degrees along the rescuer's forearm and ensure head and neck are stabilized. For a larger infant, place facedown on the rescuer's lap with head firmly supported and held lower than the trunk.
3. Administer four back blows rapidly between the shoulder blades using the heel of the hand.
4. If no relief, turn the infant over and place on a firm surface. Deliver four rapid chest thrusts over the breastbone using two fingers.
5. If no relief, open the infant's mouth by grasping the tongue and jaw between the fingers and lifting up. By removing the tongue from the back of the throat it may be possible to visualize the object and remove with a finger. If no object is seen, blindly trying to remove the obstruction with a finger may lodge it further and should be avoided.
6. If there is no breathing, give two breaths by mouth-to-mouth or mouth-to-nose resuscitation and continue these maneuvers while waiting for an ambulance.

TECHNIQUE IF THE VICTIM IS A SMALL CHILD OLDER THAN I YEAR:

1. Call an ambulance.
2. Administer the Heimlich maneuver. This requires the child to be placed on his back on a table or the floor. Place the heel of one hand in the midline between the belly button and rib cage. Next place the other hand over the first and deliver six to ten inward and upward thrusts. This should be done gently in small children.
3. If no relief, open the mouth by grasping the tongue and the lower jaw between the fingers and lifting up. If you can see the object, attempt to dislodge it; do not attempt blindly.
4. If the child is not breathing, give two breaths by mouth-to-mouth resuscitation and repeat the maneuvers above.

BROCCOLI RISOTTO

I cup arborio rice

2 cups broccoli florets, washed

2 I/2 cups Salt-Free Chicken Stock
    (recipe, page 76)

I tbsp olive oil

I/2 onion, diced

I cup (4 oz) grated Parmesan
    cheese

I tbsp salt-free butter

• Rinse rice and set aside.

• In saucepan, blanch broccoli in boiling chicken stock for 4 to 5 minutes; remove broccoli with a slotted spoon and set stock aside. (This preserves nutrients that would otherwise be lost.) Once cool, chop broccoli into baby-bite-size pieces.

• Meanwhile, in frying pan, heat oil over medium heat; sauté onion until translucent, about 5 minutes. Add rice and 1/4 cup chicken stock and cook. As the rice becomes dry, add chicken stock, keeping the rice moist; stir after each addition. Chicken stock should be added in small increments throughout the entire cooking process, 20 to 25 minutes.

• During the last 5 minutes of cooking time, add broccoli and stir gently.

• When rice is cooked it should be just tender. (Do not be tempted to add extra chicken stock, as it will cause the rice to clump.) Once cooked, remove from heat and stir in cheese and butter. Allow to cool.

• Fill ice cube trays and freeze.

• *Tip:* For younger babies you may choose to pulse risotto in food processor to achieve desired consistency.

Yield: 16 cubes

PAVAROTTI AND PASTA

Ambience may be as important as the food itself when it comes to a toddler's appetite. Make an effort to eat together as a family, and try to maintain a pleasant atmosphere throughout mealtime. This takes the focus off the toddler and reduces his temptation to refuse the meal. Peaceful dinner music may also help the toddler to see mealtime as a relaxing, positive experience.

QUICK AND EASY PASTA AND CHEESE

This simple recipe is a healthy alternative to store-bought macaroni and cheese.

1/4 cup (2 oz) cooked pasta
1/3 cup (1.5 oz) grated cheddar
    cheese
1 tbsp breast milk or formula
    (3.25% milk after age 12
    months)

• In saucepan over low heat, stir together pasta, cheese and milk. Mix until cheese melts and pasta is thoroughly coated.
• In blender or food processor, pulse the mixture to desired consistency.

Yield: 1 serving

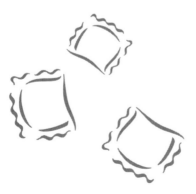

TINY TOT'S TUNA PASTA

The sauce for this recipe can be either pre-mixed with pasta, or frozen separately and mixed before serving.

1 tbsp olive oil
1/4 onion, diced
1 tbsp tomato paste
1 can (14 oz) diced tomatoes
1 can (6 oz) light tuna, drained
1 tbsp chopped fresh parsley
    (optional)
1 1/2 cups (12 oz) dried pasta,
    cooked

• In frying pan, sauté onions in oil over medium heat until translucent, about 5 minutes. Add tomato paste and tomatoes. Mix well; cover with lid and simmer for 5 minutes.
• Add tuna and stir; continue to simmer, stirring occasionally, for another 20 minutes.
• Add parsley (if using); stir.
• In blender or food processor, purée pasta and tomato mixture to desired consistency.
• Fill ice cube trays and freeze.

Yield: 16 to 18 cubes

CHICKEN AND VEGETABLE RISOTTO

1 cup arborio rice

2 tbsp olive oil

1 chicken breast, minced in food processor (or 1/2 lb ground chicken)

1/2 onion, diced

1 small carrot, washed, peeled and grated

2 stalks celery, washed, trimmed and diced

2 1/2 cups Salt-Free Chicken Stock (recipe, page 76)

1 cup (4 oz) grated Parmesan cheese

1 tbsp chopped fresh parsley (optional)

• Rinse rice and set aside.
• In frying pan, heat 1 tbsp oil over medium heat; sauté chicken until there are no traces of pink, 5 to 6 minutes. Set chicken aside.
• Using the same pan, sauté onion, carrot and celery in remaining tbsp of oil until onion is translucent, about 5 minutes.
• Add rice and 1/4 cup chicken stock; cook over medium heat. As rice becomes dry, slowly add chicken stock, keeping the rice moist and stirring after each addition. After 10 minutes the chicken should be mixed into the rice. Chicken stock should be added in small increments throughout the entire cooking process, 20 to 25 minutes. When rice is cooked it should be just tender.
• During the last 2 minutes of cooking time, add cheese and parsley (if using). Stir until cheese melts. (Do not be tempted to add extra chicken stock, as it will cause risotto to clump.) Remove from heat.
• Add parsley (if using); stir. Allow to cool.
• Fill ice cube trays and freeze.
• *Tip:* For younger babies you may choose to use a blender or food processor to purée risotto to desired consistency before freezing.

Yield: 16 to 18 cubes

CHICKPEAS AU GRATIN

I tbsp olive oil

1/2 onion, diced

I can (14 oz) chopped tomatoes

1/4 cup water

I can (19 oz) chickpeas, drained
and rinsed

2 cups broccoli florets, washed
and cut in baby-bite-size
pieces

1/3 cup (1.5 oz) grated cheddar
cheese

I tbsp chopped fresh basil
(optional)

• In frying pan, heat oil over medium heat; sauté onion until translucent, about 5 minutes. Add tomatoes, water, chickpeas and broccoli; increase heat and bring to a boil. Reduce heat and simmer, partially covered, 20 minutes. Remove from heat.

• Add cheese and basil (if using), and stir until cheese is thoroughly melted. Mash with fork.

• Fill ice cube trays and freeze.

Yield: 18 to 20 cubes

Yogurt Smoothies and Desserts

Although called "Yogurt Smoothies and Desserts" the following recipes can be served on their own as a snack or an accompaniment to any meal.

MIXED BERRY MASH

If your baby struggles with the texture of this purée, you may want to push it through a sieve to remove the seeds.

4 cups mixed frozen berries

• In saucepan, cook berries over medium heat for 15 minutes.
• With handheld immersion blender or food processor, purée berries.
• Pour into ice cube trays and freeze.

Yield: 10 to 12 cubes

MIXED BERRY YOGURT

I cube Mixed Berry Mash (recipe, page 145)
1/4 cup Balkan-style yogurt (above 3% milk fat)

• Defrost cube of Mixed Berry Mash.
• In a small bowl, combine Mixed Berry Mash and yogurt.

Yield: 1 serving

DRIED FRUIT YOGURT

Dried Fruit Purée has a rather strong flavor, so mixing it with yogurt makes it more palatable.

I cube Dried Fruit Purée (recipe, page 72)

1/3 cup high-fat (above 3%) plain yogurt

CARIBBEAN-STYLE COTTAGE CHEESE

Cottage cheese mixes well with other fruits. Try it with either grated apple or mashed banana.

2 slices papaya, washed and skin removed

1/3 cup cottage cheese

• Defrost cube of Dried Fruit Purée.

• In small bowl, combine Dried Fruit Purée and yogurt. Serve at room temperature.

Yield: 1 serving

• In small bowl, mash papaya with fork. Mix cottage cheese with fruit, and serve.

Yield: 1 serving

TROPICAL SMOOTHIE

I slice mango, washed, skin
    removed
1/3 banana, skin removed
2 tbsp high-fat (above 3%) plain
    yogurt
I tbsp unsweetened apple juice
    (approx)

• In small bowl, mash mango
and banana with fork. Using
blender or food processor, purée
fruit, yogurt and juice. Serve
immediately, before the banana
turns brown.

Yield: 1 serving

AVOCADO SMOOTHIE

1/3 avocado, washed, pit and skin
    removed
1/3 cup high-fat (above 3%) plain
    yogurt

• In small bowl, mash avocado with fork. Mix with yogurt;
serve.

Yield: 1 serving

FRUIT SMOOTHIE

This recipe can be made with
either mashed banana or any of
your baby's favorite fruit purées.

I cube fruit purée
1/3 cup high-fat (above 3%) plain
    yogurt
I tbsp unsweetened apple juice
    (approx)

• Defrost fruit purée; mix with
yogurt. If the mixture seems too
thick, add unsweetened apple
juice 1 tsp at a time until desired
consistency is reached.

Yield: 1 serving

147

Breakfast Ideas

Commercial baby cereals are the best choice for baby's breakfast, and should form the staple of the diet in the first year because they are heavily fortified with iron. It is advisable to serve commercial baby cereal well into the second year of life and until baby has a reliable intake of iron from other sources. At 8 to 10 months of age, baby can be introduced to alternative breakfast cereals for occasional variety; however, they should not replace baby cereal. Look for toddler cereals that are iron-fortified and help to promote self-feeding skills. The vast majority of adult cereals, including the ones whose names "sound" healthy, have excessive sugar and salt.

BANANA CRUNCH

Cornflakes contain traces of soybeans and therefore should not be consumed by babies suspected of having a soy allergy.

1/3 cup cornflakes
1/3 banana, skin removed
1 tbsp high-fat (above 3%) plain
    yogurt
1/4 cup breast milk or formula
    (3.25% milk after age 12 months)

• In bowl, mash cornflakes and banana together with fork. Add yogurt and enough milk to achieve desired consistency.

Yield: 1 serving

YOGURT APPLE CEREAL

Nutrios are specifically designed for babies and can be found in the baby food section of many supermarkets. If your grocery store does not carry Nutrios, Cheerios can be substituted in the following recipes.

You can make this with any of the fruit purées, or with mashed banana.

1/4 cup Nutrios or Cheerios

2 cubes apple purée (recipe, page 44)

1/3 cup high-fat (above 3%) plain yogurt

• In bowl, crush cereal with a fork.
• Defrost 2 cubes apple purée. Mix with cereal and yogurt. Serve.

Yield: 1 serving

BALANCING FIBER

Increasing fiber is a main principle in reducing fat intake and preventing both heart and bowel disease in adults. In babies less than 2 years of age, however, promoting an excessively high-fiber diet may be detrimental. Babies depend on a large intake of fats as the primary source of energy for rapid growth and brain development. Since fiber acts as a bulking agent, excessively high intakes may result in decreased intake of other food groups, most importantly fats. A healthy approach to fiber intake for your baby is several servings per week of a variety of fruits, whole grains and legumes. After 2 years of age fiber intake should be increased.

DRIED FRUIT CEREAL

1/4 cup Nutrios or Cheerios
I cube mixed Dried Fruit Purée
    (recipe, page 72)
1/3 cup high-fat (above 3%) plain
    yogurt

• In bowl, crush cereal with fork.
• Defrost 1 cube Dried Fruit Purée. Mix with cereal and yogurt. Serve.

Yield: 1 serving

BANANA PORRIDGE

This recipe can also be made with water if you don't have formula or breast milk on hand.

1/4 cup instant porridge oats
1/2 cup breast milk or formula
    (3.25% milk after age 12
    months)
1/3 banana, skin removed and
    mashed

• In saucepan, combine oats and milk over medium heat; simmer for 5 minutes, stirring occasionally.
• Mix with mashed banana. If consistency is too thick, add extra milk as needed. Serve.

Yield: 1 serving

APPLE PORRIDGE

This recipe can also be made with water if you don't have formula or breast milk on hand.

1/4 cup instant porridge oats
1/2 cup breast milk or formula
    (3.25% milk after age 12
    months)
1/2 apple, washed, peeled and
    grated

• In saucepan, combine oats, milk and apple over medium heat; simmer for 5 minutes, stirring occasionally. If consistency is too thick, add extra milk as needed. Serve.

Yield: 1 serving

MANAGING GASTROENTERITIS

At some point your child may experience diarrhea and vomiting and be diagnosed with gastroenteritis, as most children under age 3 have at least one episode per year. Gastroenteritis refers to an infection of the gastrointestinal tract, which results in diarrhea, vomiting, decreased appetite and possibly fever. By far the most common cause of gastroenteritis is viral, resulting in mild symptoms of diarrhea and vomiting without serious dehydration or illness. The exception is Rotavirus, which may cause more severe symptoms with fever and marked dehydration. Other causes of gastroenteritis are bacterial, often acquired from infected food or water, or giardia. Bacterial infections may result in blood in the stool and more serious symptoms.

In general, viral and mild bacterial infections may last 5 to 10 days. During the illness it is important to keep your child well hydrated, something you can monitor by checking for wet diapers. Recommendations from the Canadian Paediatric Society and the American Academy of Pediatrics have re-evaluated earlier positions on milk intake. Experts now believe that milk should be continued throughout the illness and does not affect the severity or duration of diarrhea in mild to moderate cases. In rare cases temporary lactose intolerance (lasting anywhere from 3 to 10 days) may develop and diarrhea will become much worse. If this occurs, your doctor may recommend an alternative to cow's milk-based formula.

The question surrounding what to eat during the illness has been under considerable debate. In the past, doctors recommended limited diets. Today, however, the thinking is that a wide diet of breads, rice, potatoes, meat, yogurt, fruits and vegetables are better tolerated than fatty foods or foods high in sugar content such as fruit juice or soft drinks.

The most effective means of preventing spread to other family members is frequent hand washing by everyone. Consult your doctor for further advice regarding gastroenteritis or for serious symptoms such as blood in the stool, fever or persistence of symptoms. Babies under 1 year of age should be evaluated by a doctor if symptoms persist longer than 24 hours.

WEEK 1

DAY 1

Breakfast	Breast or Bottle, Sngle-Grain Baby Cereal (Rice), Mashed Banana
Mid-A.M. Snack	Avocado, Whole-Wheat Toast Strips
Lunch	Breast or Bottle, Sole, Vegetables and Cheese
Mid-P.M. Snack	Breast or Bottle
Dinner	Tuscan Tomato and Chickpeas
Before Bed	Breast or Bottle

DAY 2

Breakfast	Breast or Bottle, Baby Cereal (Mixed Grain)
Mid-A.M. Snack	Caribbean-Style Cottage Cheese
Lunch	Breast or Bottle, Minestrone, Whole-Wheat Toast Strips
Mid-P.M. Snack	Breast or Bottle
Dinner	Baja Chicken Salad, Melon
Before Bed	Breast or Bottle

DAY 3

Breakfast	Breast or Bottle, Baby Cereal (Mixed Grain), Blueberry Banana Mash
Mid-A.M. Snack	Tropical Smoothie
Lunch	Breast or Bottle, Pork and Apple Purée
Mid-P.M. Snack	Breast or Bottle
Dinner	Baby's First Scramble, Whole-Wheat Toast Strips, Peas Please
Before Bed	Breast or Bottle

DAY 4

Breakfast	Breast or Bottle, Single-Grain Baby Cereal (Rice), Mashed Pear
Mid-A.M. Snack	Peeled Apple Slices
Lunch	Breast or Bottle, Spinach and Cheese, Yogurt
Mid-P.M. Snack	Breast or Bottle
Dinner	Sole with Salsa & Cheese, Mashed Banana
Before Bed	Breast or Bottle

DAY 5

Breakfast	Breast or Bottle, Single-Grain Baby Cereal (Rice), Mashed Papaya
Mid-A.M. Snack	Whole-Wheat Toast Strips, Cheese Slices
Lunch	Breast or Bottle, Lasagna Mash, Banana
Mid-P.M. Snack	Breast or Bottle
Dinner	Vichyssoise, Melon
Before Bed	Breast or Bottle

WEEK I continued

DAY 6

Breakfast	Breast or Bottle, Egg and Avocado Mash, Whole-Wheat Toast Strips
Mid-A.M. Snack	Yogurt mixed with Single-Grain Baby Cereal (Rice)
Lunch	Breast or Bottle, Shepherd's Mash
Mid-P.M. Snack	Breast or Bottle
Dinner	Baked Tomato and Zucchini au Gratin, Apple Slices
Before Bed	Breast or Bottle

DAY 7

Breakfast	Breast or Bottle, Single-Grain Baby Cereal (Rice), Apple
Mid-A.M. Snack	Fruit Smoothie
Lunch	Breast or Bottle, Broccoli Risotto, Pear Slices
Mid-P.M. Snack	Breast or Bottle
Dinner	Brown Rice and Vegetables, Melon
Before Bed	Breast or Bottle

SAMPLE DAILY MEAL PLANNER: FROM NINE TO TWELVE MONTHS

WEEK 2

DAY I

Breakfast	Breast or Bottle, Single-Grain Baby Cereal (Rice)
Mid-A.M. Snack	Whole-Wheat Toast Strips dipped in Florets and Cheese Sauce
Lunch	Breast or Bottle, Navy Beans, Yogurt
Mid-P.M. Snack	Breast or Bottle
Dinner	Maxwell's Minted Lamb, Steamed Vegetable Sticks
Before Bed	Breast or Bottle

DAY 2

Breakfast	Breast or Bottle, Baby Cereal (Mixed Grain), Mashed Pear
Mid-A.M. Snack	Melon
Lunch	Breast or Bottle, Chicken Noodle Stew, Yogurt
Mid-P.M. Snack	Breast or Bottle
Dinner	Vegetable Barley Risotto, Banana
Before Bed	Breast or Bottle

WEEK 2 continued

DAY 3

Breakfast	Breast or Bottle, Baby Cereal (Mixed Grain)
Mid-A.M. Snack	Steamed Vegetable Sticks
Lunch	Breast or Bottle, Shepherd's Mash, Blueberry Purée
Mid-P.M. Snack	Breast or Bottle
Dinner	Tuna Salad, Banana
Before Bed	Breast or Bottle

DAY 4

Breakfast	Breast or Bottle, Baby Cereal (Mixed Grain)
Mid-A.M. Snack	Down Under Fruit Salad
Lunch	Breast or Bottle, Red Snapper Salsa Provençal
Mid-P.M. Snack	Breast or Bottle
Dinner	Spinach and Cheese, Liz's Couscous
Before Bed	Breast or Bottle

DAY 5

Breakfast	Breast or Bottle, Baby Cereal (Mixed Grain)
Mid-A.M. Snack	Fruit Smoothie
Lunch	Breast or Bottle, Thanksgiving Dinner
Mid-P.M. Snack	Breast or Bottle
Dinner	Minestrone, Papaya
Before Bed	Breast or Bottle

DAY 6

Breakfast	Breast or Bottle, Single-Grain Baby Cereal (Oats), Mashed Pear
Mid-A.M. Snack	Mango Tofu Mash
Lunch	Breast or Bottle, Green Lentils, Whole-Wheat Toast Strips
Mid-P.M. Snack	Breast or Bottle
Dinner	Baby Chicken, Yogurt
Before Bed	Breast or Bottle

DAY 7

Breakfast	Breast or Bottle, Yogurt mixed with Baby Cereal (Mixed Grain)
Mid-A.M. Snack	Steamed Vegetable Sticks
Lunch	Breast or Bottle, Okanagan Summer Chicken, Banana
Mid-P.M. Snack	Breast or Bottle
Dinner	West Coast Salmon
Before Bed	Breast or Bottle

Toddlers

In your child's second year of life, you will find it important to adapt to her individual appetite. Meeting these requirements may mean frequent feedings throughout the day; your child may require four to six feedings in addition to milk intake. At this stage the goal is to provide nutritious food from all four food groups.

The statement of the Joint Working Group of the Canadian Paediatric Society, Dietitians of Canada, and Health Canada recommends small, frequent, energy-dense feedings. For now, put aside the idea of three square meals a day and respect your toddler's hunger and willingness to eat. Appetite varies according to growth, activity, fatigue, frustration, illness and social setting. Toddlers should be given the opportunity to ask for more if they are hungry and to say "enough" when they are not.

At this stage the goal is to encourage your toddler to participate in family meals as often as possible. Research tells us that the modeling of good eating habits is one of the best ways to instill healthy eating habits in your children. Many parents find their toddlers are ready for table foods, while others find success with meals made up of finger foods. And many babies of this age continue to enjoy mushy purées. It is not uncommon for toddlers to advance from preferring mashed carrots one week to soft-cooked carrot sticks the next. If your child refuses a meal, try not to get frustrated. Take the meal away and offer a snack later. Avoid the temptation to focus on the intake of a single meal. Instead, evaluate your toddler's nutritional intake over several days to weeks. It is important to be flexible and sensitive to changing preferences. Patience and a sense of humor are vital; this can be a frustrating time for all.

When out and about, your toddler does not have to subsist on a diet of convenience food. With a little preparation he can enjoy healthy snacks and meals all day long. Whole-wheat toast strips, whole-grain crackers, cereal, rice crackers, steamed vegetable sticks, fruit and pieces of shredded cheese can be easily packed in airtight containers. Bring a cup and a non-BPA bottle containing water. On a hot day, freeze the bottle before leaving; this will help to keep the food cool, and the drink will melt as the day progresses.

Creative (and sometimes silly!) presentation is effective. Drawing a funny face on a bowl of porridge can be a hit with fussy eaters, or, instead of sprinkling berries on a bowl of cereal, arrange them into a happy face. Food decorating can add pizzazz to any meal. For example, slices of hard-boiled eggs, cherry tomatoes and olives make wonderful eyes. Steamed broccoli florets become a wild head of hair. A steamed carrot stick becomes the nose, and slices of apple or orange form the mouth. Toddlers delight in eating these funny faces. Be imaginative!

Many of the following recipes are designed to be made in bulk and frozen in airtight containers. This method facilitates the serving of convenient, individual toddler meals. For these recipes you will need five or six small, freezer-safe, airtight containers, or you can use muffin tins covered with tin foil or parchment paper.

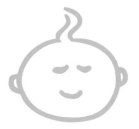

VEGETABLE RAGOUT

Vegetable Ragout is a great meal for the entire family and a yummy way to entice your toddler to eat her veggies. This pasta sauce is designed to be made in bulk and frozen in either small airtight containers or ice cube trays.

1/2 onion, cut in half

2 carrots, washed, trimmed and
    sliced

2 stalks celery, washed, trimmed
    and sliced

8 broccoli florets, washed

2 cloves garlic (whole)

I tbsp dried oregano

2 tbsp olive oil

I 1/2 lb ground beef

I can (5.5 oz) tomato paste

3 cans (each 14 oz) diced toma-
    toes

I bay leaf (optional)

1/2 cup chopped fresh basil
    (optional)

Parmesan cheese

• In blender or food processor, finely chop onion, carrots, celery, broccoli, garlic and oregano.
• In frying pan, heat oil over medium heat; sauté finely chopped vegetables for 10 minutes.
• Crumble in ground beef and cook until no longer pink. Add tomato paste, stirring until mixture is thoroughly coated.
• Add tomatoes and bay leaf (if using); stir. Bring to a rapid boil, reduce heat and simmer for 45 minutes, stirring occasionally. During the last 10 minutes of cooking time, add basil (if using) and stir.
• Remove bay leaf and allow stew to cool. Pour into airtight containers or ice cube trays and freeze.
• *To serve:* Defrost in refrigerator, heat, pour over cooked pasta and sprinkle with Parmesan cheese to taste.

Yield: 5 to 6 small airtight containers

YUMMY CHICKEN FINGERS

Homemade chicken fingers are a tasty and healthy alternative to store-bought, which often contain additives and preservatives. Serve with homemade Tomato Sauce (recipe, page 124) or one of your baby's favorite vegetable purées. These fingers work equally well with or without cheese; however, cheese does add zest.

1/2 chicken breast

2 cups whole-wheat bread crumbs (recipe, page 159)

1/2 cup (2 oz) grated Parmesan cheese (optional)

2 eggs, beaten

1 tbsp olive oil

• Cut chicken breast across the width into 8 fingers.
• In plastic bag, combine bread crumbs and cheese (if using).
• Dip chicken fingers into beaten eggs. Place fingers in bag, one at a time, and shake until thoroughly coated with bread crumbs.

• Spread oil on baking sheet. Place chicken fingers on sheet and bake in 350°F oven for 10 minutes. Flip chicken and bake for another 10 to 12 minutes. When cooked, chicken fingers should be crispy and golden brown.
• *Tip:* This recipe can be made in bulk and frozen in either air-tight containers or freezer bags. To make in bulk, double the recipe and freeze before baking.
• *To serve:* Defrost in refrigerator. Cook as above.

Yield: 8 chicken fingers

WHOLE-WHEAT BREAD CRUMBS

8 slices whole-wheat bread

• Lightly toast bread. Remove from toaster and allow to stand for 5 minutes until bread is dry.
• Pulse in food processor until crumbs are a fine consistency.

Yield: 2 cups (approx)

159

COPING WITH THE PICKY TODDLER

Although frustrating for parents and caregivers, selective or picky eating is something most toddlers and preschoolers do naturally. Babies tend to have a relatively good acceptance of new foods, but as many children progress through the toddler years they become choosier in terms of both quantity and selection. This is due in part to a relative slowing of the rate at which they are growing. In the first year your baby will triple her birth weight. If she continued to gain at this rate she would weigh around 200 pounds by the time she reached the age of 3!

Sometimes how quickly a child moves through a fussy stage depends on how it is handled. Don't force or pressure your child to eat something she doesn't like. The goal is not "one more bite," but rather to raise a healthy eater. This means encouraging your child to listen to her body's cues and to stop eating when she is full. A healthy baby comes into this world instinctively knowing when to turn her head away, indicating she has had enough. As children grow, some lose touch with these cues and overeat when given the chance. In a world where childhood obesity is on the rise, how much sense does it make to force kids to eat? Resist the temptation to use dessert as a reward—this isn't a pattern you want to establish since it can lead to a preference for sweeter foods.

Do not decide your child dislikes fish because it has been rejected once or even a few times. Instead, continue to offer it in a relaxed environment. It often takes as many as ten to twenty exposures before a new food is accepted. The development of healthy life-long eating habits takes perseverance and dedication, but these habits may have an enduring impact on your child's future health.

Make an effort to ensure portions are small and realistic. There is nothing more off-putting to a toddler than a large portion of unfamiliar food. When introducing a new food, serve a small taste alongside a familiar favorite.

Encourage physical activity, as there is nothing like a little exercise to build up the appetite. If you are still concerned about your toddler's appetite, evaluate her juice and milk consumption. Excess milk and/or juice consumption can negatively impact the appetite. If your child is still drinking out of a bottle, switch her to a cup. The change will likely cause her to drink less and eat more.

Be reassured that no healthy toddler will starve herself and in most cases she is eating what she needs to thrive. If your worries persist, see your doctor, who will measure your child's growth and calculate her body mass index (BMI) to ensure she is not underweight. And remember that the vast majority of finicky toddlers grow into food-loving adults!

BABY BEEFCAKES

I lb ground beef

I egg

I medium potato, baked

I small carrot, washed, peeled and finely grated

I tbsp chopped fresh parsley (optional)

I tbsp tomato paste

2 tbsp onion, finely diced

I tbsp olive oil

• In large bowl, mix all ingredients except olive oil thoroughly. Shape into small patties.

• Spread oil on baking sheet. Place patties on sheet and flatten with fork. Bake in 350°F oven for 10 minutes on each side.

• Allow to cool; freeze in freezer bags.

• *To serve:* Defrost in refrigerator. Heat in 350°F oven until warm.

Yield: 18 patties

IS MY CHILD TOO OLD FOR A BOTTLE?

In an ideal world your baby would go from the breast to the cup, but for many families this simply isn't feasible. The World Health Organization recommends that the bottle be taken away after 15 months. However, the bottle is often a great source of comfort for toddlers and the thought of giving it up often fills both parents and children with dread.

The problem with the bottle is that there is a tendency for children to consume a disproportionate amount of their daily calories through it. These children usually drink more milk, which is nutritionally incomplete and very low in iron, at the expense of eating other foods; iron deficiency and anemia can result. Furthermore, children who have unfettered access to the bottle often develop dental caries. These cavities are the result of the teeth continually being bathed in lactose, the sugar naturally present in milk.

During the second year of life your baby should go from drinking a maximum of around 3 cups (24 oz) of milk per day to only 2 cups (16 oz) of milk per day by his second birthday. Ideally this happens gradually, and often giving up the bottle helps facilitate the process. If you are reluctant to give up the bottle "cold turkey," start slowly, by removing the least favorite bottle first. It is best to start the withdrawal process when things are stable at home and not, for instance, when you are traveling or dealing with illness or the arrival of a new sibling. After the age of 2, 2 cups of milk a day is sufficient.

HALIBUT FISH STICKS

Halibut fish sticks are a healthy alternative to commercial fish sticks and can be made with any white fish. These fish sticks work equally well with or without cheese; however, cheese does contribute both flavor and added protein.

8 oz halibut, skin and bones
    removed
2 cups whole-wheat bread
    crumbs (recipe, page 159)
1/2 cup (2 oz) grated Parmesan
    cheese (optional)
2 eggs, beaten
1 tbsp olive oil

• Cut fish into 8 sticks, remembering to look carefully for any remaining bones.
• In plastic bag, combine bread crumbs and cheese (if using).
• Dip fish sticks into beaten eggs. Place sticks in bag, one at a time, and shake until thoroughly coated with bread crumbs.
• Spread oil on baking sheet. Place fish sticks on sheet and bake in 350°F oven for 10 minutes. Flip fish and bake for another 10 minutes. When ready, fish sticks should be crispy and golden brown.
• *Tip:* This recipe can be made in bulk and frozen in either airtight containers or freezer bags. To make in bulk, double recipe and freeze before baking.
• *To serve:* Defrost in refrigerator. Cook as above.

Yield: 8 fish sticks

GOURMET TUNA MELTS

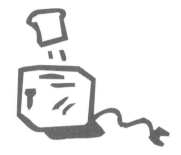

This recipe makes a wholesome lunch for the whole family. If only serving baby, make just 1 tuna melt.

I can (6 oz) light tuna, drained
I tbsp lemon juice
I tbsp red onion, finely diced
I tbsp chopped fresh dill
2 tbsp mayonnaise
4 slices whole-wheat bread
4 oz cheddar cheese, thinly sliced

• In bowl, thoroughly combine tuna, lemon juice, onion, dill and mayonnaise.
• Turn oven temperature to broil. Lightly toast bread in oven (to prevent bread from becoming soggy when broiled with tuna).
• Spread toast with tuna and cheese, and place on baking sheet. Broil in 400°F oven about 2 minutes or until cheese begins to bubble.
• Allow to cool. Remove crusts and cut in bite-size pieces to serve.

Yield: 4 tuna melts

CRISPY TUNA BALLS

This recipe is designed to be made in bulk and frozen. Individual portions can then be defrosted and baked.

I medium potato, baked
I egg, beaten
I can (6 oz) light tuna, drained
I tbsp red onion, finely diced
2 cups whole-wheat bread
    crumbs (recipe, page 159)
I tbsp olive oil

• Cut potato in half and scoop out the inside. In blender or food processor, combine potato, egg, tuna and onion.
• Pour bread crumbs into plastic bag.
• Scoop 1 tbsp of tuna mince and form into ball. Place ball in bag and shake until thoroughly coated with bread crumbs.

• Place tuna balls in airtight freezer bags and freeze.

• *To serve:* Defrost tuna balls in refrigerator. Spread oil on baking sheet. Place tuna balls on sheet and bake in 350°F oven for 10 minutes. Flip and bake for another 10 minutes. When cooked, tuna balls should be crispy and golden brown.

Yield: 16 to 18 balls

CRISPY B.C. SALMON BALLS

This recipe is designed to be made in bulk and frozen. Individual portions can then be defrosted and baked.

I medium potato, baked

I egg, beaten

10 oz salmon, skin and bones removed, cut in cubes

I tsp chopped fresh dill (optional)

Dash lemon juice

I tbsp onion, finely diced

2 cups whole-wheat bread crumbs (recipe, page 159)

2 tbsp olive oil

• Cut potato in half and scoop out the inside. In blender or food processor, combine potato, egg, salmon, dill (if using), lemon juice and onion.

• Pour bread crumbs into plastic bag.

• Scoop 1 tbsp of salmon mince and form into ball. Place ball in bag and shake until thoroughly coated with bread crumbs.

• Place salmon balls in airtight freezer bags and freeze.

• *To serve:* Defrost salmon balls in refrigerator. Spread oil on baking sheet. Place salmon balls on sheet and bake in 350°F oven for 10 minutes. Flip and bake for another 10 minutes. When done, salmon balls should be crispy and golden brown.

Yield: 16 to 18 balls

FRITTATA

2 potatoes, washed, peeled and
  cut in cubes
I tbsp salt-free butter
10 eggs, beaten

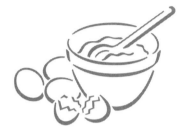

• In saucepan of boiling water, parboil potatoes for 5 to 10 minutes, just until tender but not cooked through.

• In frying pan over medium heat, heat butter and sauté potatoes for 10 minutes. Add eggs, and mix thoroughly.

• Pour egg mixture into greased 8" x 8" baking dish. Bake in 400°F oven for about 30 to 40 minutes, or until frittata is golden brown around the edges and just firm to touch. If in doubt, insert a knife into the middle; it should come out clean.

Yield: 6 servings

WHAT ARE OMEGA-3 EGGS?

As little as 2 to 3 servings of fish per week is thought to reduce the risk of heart disease and stroke in adults, and, when included in the maternal diet, it can enhance newborn brain and retinal development. Recently, omega-3 eggs have been developed that contain 300 to 500 times more omega-3 than regular eggs. Researchers fed hens a diet of marine algae, which is the source of omega-3 for the marine food chain and the reason for the high quantity of omega-3 in fish. Consuming one omega-3 egg is equivalent to consuming I serving of fish.

THE SCRAMBLER

I tbsp salt-free butter

4 eggs

1/3 cup (1.5 oz) grated cheddar
    cheese

I tomato, skinned and diced (see
    Skinned Seeded Tomatoes,
    page 124)

I tbsp chopped fresh basil
    (optional)

• In frying pan, melt butter
over low heat.
• In bowl, thoroughly whisk
eggs and cheese together and
add mixture to pan. Scramble
eggs until cooked.
• Remove from heat. Add tomato and basil (if using); stir until
combined.

Yield: 2 servings

PIZZA SOLDIERS

I slice whole-wheat bread

I tsp tomato paste

1/4 cup (I oz) grated mozzarella
    cheese

• Lightly toast bread.
• Thinly spread tomato paste
on toast and top with cheese.
• Broil about 2 minutes or until
cheese melts.
• Remove crust and cut in strips.

Yield: 1 serving

CHICKEN POTPIE

2 tbsp olive oil

1/2 onion, diced

2 stalks celery, washed, trimmed
   and diced

1 tbsp chopped fresh tarragon
   (optional)

10 mushrooms, thinly sliced

1 lb minced chicken

1 1/2 cups low-sodium or Salt-Free
   Chicken Stock (recipe, page 76)

2 carrots, washed, peeled and cut
   in bite-size pieces

1 cup broccoli florets, washed

1 tbsp chopped fresh parsley
   (optional)

4 large potatoes, washed, peeled
   and chopped

1/2 cup (3.25%) milk

4 tbsp salt-free butter

• In large frying pan, heat 1 tbsp oil over medium heat; sauté onion, celery and tarragon (if using) for 5 minutes. Add remaining tbsp of oil and mushrooms; continue to sauté, stirring occasionally, for 15 minutes. Stir in minced chicken; continue to sauté for 10 minutes.

• Add chicken stock, carrots and broccoli; bring to a boil. Reduce heat and simmer until vegetables are tender, stirring occasionally.

• Remove from heat. Add parsley (if using); stir.

• In pot of salted, boiling water, cook potatoes until tender. Drain well; mash with milk and butter. Spread a layer of chicken mixture in each of 5 or 6 small airtight containers. Top with potato. Freeze.

• *To serve:* Defrost in refrigerator. Bake in 350°F oven until pie is bubbling around the edges, 20 to 25 minutes. Dotting pie with butter and broiling for last 2 minutes of cooking time will make the topping golden brown and crispy.

Yield: 5 to 6 small containers

SHEPHERD'S PIE

1 tbsp olive oil

1/2 onion, diced

1 stalk celery, washed, trimmed
and diced

1 lb ground beef

1 carrot, washed, peeled and cut
in bite-size pieces

1 cup canned whole-kernel corn,
rinsed and drained

1 can (14 oz) diced tomatoes

4 tbsp tomato paste

1 tbsp chopped fresh parsley,
(optional)

4 large potatoes, washed, peeled
and chopped

1/2 cup (3.25%) milk

4 tbsp salt-free butter

• In frying pan, heat oil over low heat; sauté onion and celery until onion is translucent, about 5 minutes. Add beef and sauté until it is no longer pink, about 10 minutes.

• Add carrot, corn, tomatoes, tomato paste and parsley (if using); mix thoroughly. Simmer, partially covered, until carrots are tender, about 25 minutes.

• In pot of salted, boiling water, cook potato until tender. Drain well; mash with milk and butter. Spread a layer of meat in each of 5 or 6 small airtight containers. Top with potato. Freeze.

• *To serve:* Defrost in refrigerator. Bake in 350°F oven until pie is bubbling around the edges, 20 to 25 minutes. Dotting pie with butter and broiling for last 2 minutes of cooking time will make the topping golden brown and crispy.

Yield: 5 to 6 small containers

FISH PIE

I lb halibut or other white fish,
   skin and bones removed

I bay leaf

2 1/2 cups (3.25%) milk

2 carrots, washed, peeled and cut
   in bite-size pieces

I tbsp butter

I tbsp flour (approx)

I 1/2 cups (6 oz) grated cheddar
   cheese, firmly packed

4 hard-boiled eggs, crumbled

I tbsp chopped fresh chives
   (optional)

4 large potatoes, washed, peeled
   and chopped

4 tbsp salt-free butter

• Cut fish into cubes. Place in saucepan with bay leaf; cover with 2 cups of milk. Bring to a light boil; reduce heat and simmer until fish flakes, about 20 minutes. Drain fish; set poaching milk aside. Remove bay leaf. Once cool, crumble fish in bowl with fingers, checking for any remaining bones.

• In steamer, cook carrots over boiling water until tender.

• In large saucepan, whisk together butter and flour over medium heat until paste forms. Slowly add 1/2 cup of poaching milk, whisking until lumps disappear. Add both cheese and another 1/2 cup of poaching milk, whisking until cheese melts and sauce thickens.

• Once sauce is smooth and creamy, add to fish. Mix in carrots, eggs and chives (if using).

• In pot of salted, boiling water, cook potatoes until tender. Drain well; mash with the remaining 1/2 cup milk and butter. Spread a layer of fish mixture in each of 4 or 5 small airtight containers. Top with potato. Freeze.

• *To serve:* Defrost in refrigerator. Bake in 350°F until pie is bubbling around the edges, 20 to 25 minutes. Dotting pie with butter and broiling for last 2 minutes of cooking time will make the topping golden brown and crispy.

Yield: 4 to 5 small containers

PIZZA

This easy-to-make pizza is a crowd-pleaser among children of all ages. It can be made with a variety of toppings, and kids love the opportunity to make their own. Let them experiment!

1 10-inch soft flour tortilla
1 tbsp tomato paste
1/3 cup (1.5 oz) grated cheddar
  cheese
1 slice Black Forest ham, cut in
  strips

• Broil tortilla in oven until edges begin to turn golden brown, 4 to 5 minutes.
• Allow tortilla to cool; spread evenly with tomato paste. Sprinkle with cheese and ham.
• Broil in oven until cheese melts, 1 to 2 minutes.
• Allow to cool. Using scissors, cut in wedges and serve.

Yield: 1 serving

CHILDHOOD OBESITY

Childhood obesity is increasing at an alarming rate, due to a greater reliance on and availability of convenience food and a more sedentary lifestyle. There is also a known hereditary component to obesity. Although it is unnecessary and unhealthy to restrict fats for babies under 2 years old, your doctor may address dietary practices if your child exceeds upper weight limits on standardized growth curves and is considered at risk for obesity (see Appendix III, page 195). For instance, instead of focusing on the fat content of your baby's milk, your doctor may advise limiting milk intake to between 16 and 24 oz. For all children it is good practice to limit processed foods and offer fruits and vegetables for snacks. For the infant with the robust appetite offering more fruits and vegetables is recommended. Limit juice and offer water with and between meals. After 2 years, switching to 2% milk is advised. If your doctor is still concerned, she may possibly recommend switching to an even lower fat milk. It is good practice with all babies and children to avoid using food as comfort for disappointment or pain, or using fast food or sweets as a reward. After all, obesity and its health consequences are no treat.

BAKED MACARONI AND CHEESE

This dish could serve as a meal for the entire family. For smaller babies, individual portions can be pulsed in the blender or food processor until desired consistency is reached. Leftovers can be stored in the refrigerator, making convenient baby and toddler meals. Alternatively, pour the pasta and sauce mixture into airtight containers and freeze in individual portions. *To serve:* Defrost in refrigerator. Bake in 350°F oven or heat in a saucepan over low heat.

4 tbsp salt-free butter

2 tbsp flour

2 cups (3.25%) milk

3 cups grated sharp cheddar cheese, firmly packed (I lb)

I cup (4 oz) grated Parmesan cheese

4 cups macaroni

4 tbsp whole-wheat bread crumbs (recipe, page 159)

• *To make cheese sauce:* In saucepan, whisk together 2 tbsp butter and flour over medium heat. Add 1 cup of milk; continue to whisk until lumps disappear. Add cheddar cheese and remaining cup of milk, whisking until cheese melts. Stir in 1/2 cup of Parmesan cheese; allow sauce to thicken.

• Cook macaroni until al dente. Drain and mix with cheese sauce until pasta is thoroughly coated.

• Pour mixture into greased 10" x 15" baking dish.

• In saucepan, melt 2 tbsp of butter. Add bread crumbs; stir until bread crumbs are coated. Remove from heat; mix with remaining Parmesan cheese. Sprinkle bread crumbs over macaroni and cheese.

• Bake in 350°F oven until warm, 30 minutes (approx).

Yield: 1 10" x 15" baking dish (Approximately 8 to 10 Servings)

Silly Sandwich Ideas

Use cookie cutters to produce an entertaining variety of sandwich shapes and sizes. Sandwiches cut with cookie rounds can be decorated with sliced cherry tomatoes and soft-cooked carrots to become funny faces. Mix cream cheese with one of your baby's favorite purées to make a tasty sandwich filling; cream cheese mixed with apple purée, mashed avocado or mashed banana are just a few possibilities. Remember to make your sandwiches with whole-wheat bread. This is your chance to form life-long habits.

Dips

Even fussy eaters enjoy dips. The following easy-to-prepare dips make savory, nutritious snacks that can be enjoyed by the whole family. Instead of serving them with chips, try whole-wheat toast strips, whole-grain crackers or steamed vegetables.

HUMMUS

1 can (19 oz) chickpeas, drained
    and rinsed
1 tbsp olive oil
1 tbsp fresh lemon juice

• In blender or food processor, purée chickpeas, oil and lemon juice.
• Serve with toasted whole-wheat pita bread or steamed vegetables.

GUACAMOLE

1 ripe avocado, washed
1 tbsp high-fat (above 3%) plain
    yogurt
Dash lemon juice

• Cut avocado in half; remove pit and scoop out fruit.
• In small bowl, mash avocado with fork. Add yogurt and lemon juice. Mix thoroughly.
• Serve with steamed vegetables or whole-wheat toast strips.

ROASTED RED PEPPER HUMMUS

1 sweet red pepper, washed, cut
    in half lengthwise, stem and
    seeds removed
1 can (19 oz) chickpeas, drained
    and rinsed
1/3 cup high-fat (above 3%) plain
    yogurt
1 clove garlic, crushed
1 tbsp chopped fresh basil
    (optional)

• *To roast pepper:* Place pepper halves cut side down on a large sheet of tinfoil; roast in oven, 10 to 15 minutes, until the skin has bubbled and darkened. Remove from oven, wrap in foil and allow pepper to sit for 20 minutes (to enable it to continue to cook). Once pepper is cool, peel away skin.
• In blender or food processor, purée pepper, chickpeas, yogurt and garlic until smooth.
• Serve dip in a small bowl, sprinkled with basil (if using), with steamed vegetables and toasted whole-wheat pita triangles.

Baked Potatoes

Baked potatoes are a good source of both vitamin C and carbohydrates. To make the following potato recipes quickly and easily, use a microwave to bake the potato. Don't forget to prick the potato with a fork several times before microwaving. Cooking times will vary, so refer to your manufacturer's instructions.

CHEESY POTATO DELUXE

1 potato, scrubbed, blemishes removed and baked

1/3 cup high-fat (above 3%) plain yogurt

2 tbsp grated Parmesan cheese

1/2 cup (2 oz) grated cheddar cheese

5 thin slices green onion (optional)

• Cut potato in half lengthwise; scoop out flesh, leaving enough around the sides so that the potato skin keeps its shape.

• In bowl, mash potato; mix with yogurt and cheeses. Spoon the mixture back into the potato skin. Bake in 350°F oven until potato mixture is warmed through, 10 to 15 minutes. Broil for 2 minutes to make the topping crispy. Sprinkle with green onion. Serve.

Yield: 1 serving

VEGETABLE RAGOUT POTATO

I potato, scrubbed, blemishes
   removed and baked
1/3 cup Vegetable Ragout (recipe,
   page 158)
1/3 cup (1.5 oz) grated cheddar
   cheese
5 thin slices green onion
I tbsp chopped fresh basil
   (optional)

• Cut potato in half lengthwise and pour vegetable ragout over flesh; sprinkle with cheese.
• Bake in 350°F oven until cheese melts and potato is warmed through, 10 to 15 minutes. Sprinkle with green onion and basil (if using). Serve.

Yield: 1 serving

CHEESY BROCCOLI POTATO

I potato, scrubbed, blemishes
   removed and baked
3 broccoli florets, washed,
   steamed and diced
2 tbsp high-fat (above 3%) plain
   yogurt
1/3 cup (1.5 oz) grated cheddar
   cheese
5 thin slices green onion

• Cut potato in half lengthwise. Scoop out flesh, leaving enough around the sides so that the potato skin keeps its shape.
• In bowl, mash potato; mix with broccoli, yogurt and cheese. Spoon the mixture back into the potato skin. Bake in 350°F oven until potato mixture is warmed through, 10 to 15 minutes. Broil for 2 minutes to make the topping crispy. Sprinkle with green onion. Serve.

Yield: 1 serving

TODDLERS

TODDLERS

POTATO WEDGES

These potato wedges, a healthy alternative to store-bought french fries, are perfect for little hands to grasp. Serve alone, or with homemade Tomato Sauce (recipe, page 124) or your baby's favorite purée.

I baking potato, scrubbed, blemishes removed
2 tbsp olive oil

• Cut potato in half lengthwise. Segment each half into 5 to 6 sections, depending on the size of the potato.
• In bowl, toss segments with olive oil. Roast in 375°F oven for 1 hour, or until potatoes are crispy and golden.

Yield: 10 to 12 potato wedges

FRUIT SHAKE

This shake can be made with fresh fruit, but frozen berries give it a refreshing frostiness.

I cup (3.25%) milk
I banana, skin removed
1/2 cup high-fat (above 3%) plain yogurt
1/2 cup frozen mixed berries

• In blender, purée milk, banana, yogurt and berries until frothy.

Yield: 4 servings

VERY BERRY SHAKE

I cup orange juice
I banana, skin removed
1/2 cup frozen mixed berries

• In blender, purée orange juice, banana and berries until frothy.

Yield: 2 servings

Soups

Many toddlers who refuse to eat vegetables will happily eat them disguised in soup. The following recipes can be served to the whole family. All require either low-sodium or salt-free chicken stock. Low-sodium chicken stock is now conveniently available in most grocery stores, or you can make your own Salt-Free Chicken Stock (recipe, page 76).

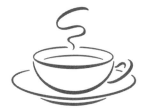

LENTIL SOUP

2 tbsp olive oil

I onion, diced

I stalk celery, washed, trimmed
and diced

2 cloves garlic, crushed

I tbsp cumin

I tsp curry powder

4 carrots, washed, peeled and
sliced

2 large potatoes, washed, peeled
and cubed

I0 cups low-sodium or Salt-Free
Chicken Stock (recipe, page 76)

I can (I4 oz) diced tomatoes

I I/3 cups dried green lentils,
rinsed and drained

I/4 cup chopped fresh cilantro
(optional)

• In large pot, heat oil over medium heat; sauté onion, celery, garlic, cumin and curry powder for 10 minutes. Add carrots, potatoes and stock; bring to a boil. Reduce heat and simmer until vegetables are tender, about 20 minutes.

• Using strainer, separate stock from vegetables; set stock aside.

• In blender or food processor, purée vegetables to a fine consistency.

• Return vegetables to pot over low heat and add stock. Add tomatoes and lentils, stir, and bring to a boil. Reduce heat and simmer, partially covered, for 1 hour.

• Remove from heat; mix in cilantro (if using). Allow to cool.

• Pour into airtight containers. Freeze.

Yield: 10 to 12 Servings

MOROCCAN VEGETABLE SOUP

3 tbsp olive oil

I onion, diced

I stalk celery, washed, trimmed and diced

I can (19 oz) chickpeas, rinsed and drained

I tbsp cumin (approx)

I clove garlic, crushed

10 cups low-sodium chicken stock or Salt-Free Chicken Stock (recipe, page 76)

I potato, washed, peeled and cubed

I cup broccoli florets, washed

4 carrots, washed, peeled and sliced

I can (14 oz) diced tomatoes

2 large handfuls spinach, washed and tough stems removed

• In large pot, heat oil over medium heat; sauté onion and celery until onion is translucent, about 5 minutes.

• Add chickpeas, cumin and garlic; continue to sauté for another 10 minutes.

• Add chicken stock, potato, broccoli, carrots and tomatoes. Bring to a rapid boil, reduce heat and simmer, partially covered, for 1 hour, stirring occasionally. Add spinach for the last 5 minutes of cooking time.

• Pour mixture through a strainer, separating stock from vegetables; set stock aside.

• In blender or food processor, purée vegetables to a rough consistency. In pot over medium heat, combine vegetables and stock.

• Allow to cool. Pour contents into airtight containers and freeze.

Yield: 10 to 12 Servings

VEGETABLE BARLEY SOUP

3 tbsp olive oil

I onion, diced

3 stalks celery, washed, trimmed
   and sliced

2 cloves garlic, crushed

10 cups low-sodium or Salt-Free
   Chicken Stock (recipe, page 76)

I can (14 oz) diced tomatoes

1/2 cup barley, rinsed and drained

3 carrots, washed, peeled and
   sliced

I potato, washed, peeled and cut
   in bite-size pieces

1/4 cup chopped fresh parsley
   (optional)

• In large pot, heat oil over medium heat; sauté onion, celery and garlic for 10 minutes.

• Add chicken stock, tomatoes and barley, and bring to a boil. Reduce heat and simmer for 30 minutes, partially covered. Stir occasionally.

• Add carrots, potato and parsley (if using). Continue to simmer until vegetables are tender, about 30 minutes.

• Allow soup to cool. Pour into airtight containers. Freeze.

• *Tip:* For younger toddlers you may choose to purée this soup with a blender or food processor before freezing.

Yield: 10 to 12 Servings

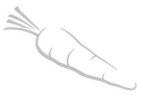

BROCCOLI SOUP

This hearty soup can also be served with grated Parmesan cheese: simply stir 2 tbsp of grated cheese into a bowl of soup, and serve.

3 tbsp olive oil

I onion, diced

8 cups low-sodium or Salt-Free
   Chicken Stock (recipe, page 76)

2 medium bunches broccoli,
   washed and cut in florets

I potato, washed, peeled and cut
   in cubes

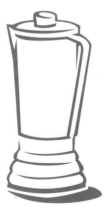

• In large pot, heat oil over medium heat; sauté onion until translucent, about 5 minutes. Add chicken stock and vegetables. Bring to rapid boil, reduce heat and simmer until vegetables are tender, about 20 to 25 minutes.

• Using strainer, separate vegetables from stock; set stock aside.

• In blender or food processor, purée vegetables to a rough consistency.

• In pot over low heat, combine puréed vegetables and stock.

• Allow soup to cool. Pour into airtight containers. Freeze.

Yield: 10 Servings

ROASTED RED PEPPER AND TOMATO SOUP

This recipe comes from Brenda's book *The Good Food Book for Families*. If you cannot find Roma tomatoes, regular ones can be substituted.

3 lb Roma tomatoes, cored and
   quartered
3 red bell peppers, halved and
   seeded
I head garlic, top removed
6 tbsp canola oil (plus an extra
   drizzle)
I onion, diced
4 carrots, grated
7 to 8 cups low-sodium or Salt-
   Free Chicken Stock (recipe,
   page 76)

• Line 2 baking sheets with tinfoil or parchment paper. Lay tomatoes and peppers on baking sheets and drizzle with 1/4 cup of oil.
• Drizzle a little more oil over garlic, wrap in foil and place on baking sheet.
• Bake tomatoes, peppers and garlic in 350°F oven for 45 minutes.
• In large pot or stockpot, heat 2 tbsp oil over medium heat; sauté onions and carrots for 10 minutes or until soft.
• Remove vegetables from oven and unwrap garlic. Once cool, squeeze garlic onto vegetables, discarding skin. The edges of the peppers will likely have blackened. If this is the case, cut these edges off and discard blackened bits.
• Add roasted vegetables to stockpot over medium heat, and sauté for another 5 minutes.
• Using handheld immersion blender, purée vegetables until smooth. If you do not have a hand blender, remove vegetables from pot and purée in a food processor or blender until smooth, then transfer vegetables back to stockpot.
• Add 7 cups of stock, mix thoroughly and bring to a boil; turn down heat and simmer for 20 minutes.
• If soup seems too thick, add extra stock until desired consistency is reached.
• Allow soup to cool. Pour into airtight containers. Freeze.

Yield: 10 Servings

Appendix I: Canada's Food Guide

Canada's new food guide is officially designed to be used by Canadians 2 years old and over. The food guide was developed to help Canadians establish a pattern of eating that meets their nutritional requirements while reducing the risk of developing chronic disease. It does so by recommending the amounts and types of foods Canadians should be eating. By the time your baby is 2 years old he should be eating 4 servings of Vegetables and Fruit, 3 servings of Grain Products, 2 servings of Milk and Alternatives and 1 serving of Meat and Alternatives per day. The easiest way to ensure he is ready to achieve this goal is to continually serve a wide variety of foods from all four food groups.

Canada's new food guide

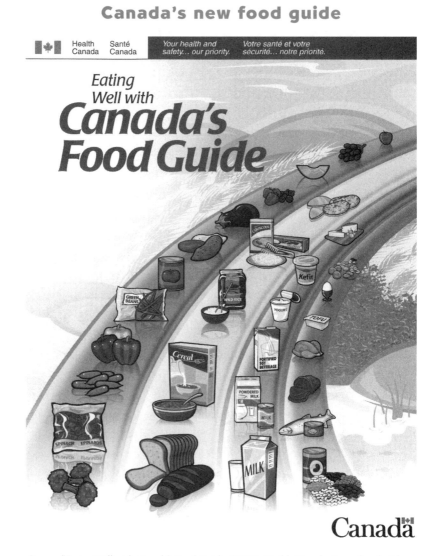

Source: "Eating Well with Canada's Food Guide, (2007), Health Canada. Reproduced with the permission of the Minister of Public Works and Government Services Canada, 2007.

Recommended Number of *Food Guide Servings* per Day

	Children			Teens		Adults			
Age in Years	2-3	4-8	9-13	14-18		19-50		51+	
Sex	Girls and Boys			Females	Males	Females	Males	Females	Males
Vegetables and Fruit	4	5	6	7	8	7-8	8-10	7	7
Grain Products	3	4	6	6	7	6-7	8	6	7
Milk and Alternatives	2	2	3-4	3-4	3-4	2	2	3	3
Meat and Alternatives	1	1	1-2	2	3	2	3	2	3

The chart above shows how many Food Guide Servings you need from each of the four food groups every day.

Having the amount and type of food recommended and following the tips in *Canada's Food Guide* will help:

• Meet your needs for vitamins, minerals and other nutrients.
• Reduce your risk of obesity, type 2 diabetes, heart disease, certain types of cancer and osteoporosis.
• Contribute to your overall health and vitality.

What is One Food Guide Serving?
Look at the examples below.

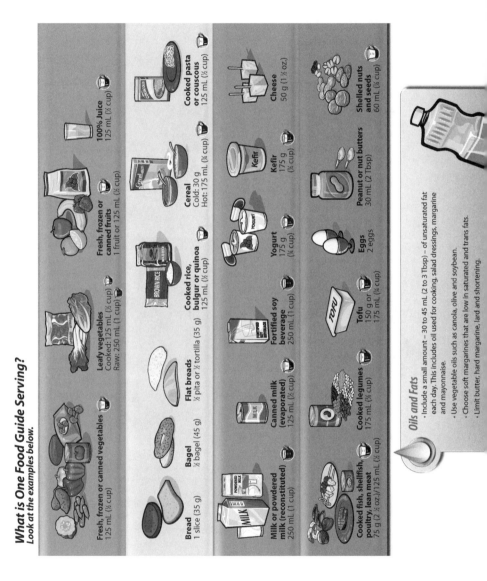

Fresh, frozen or canned vegetables
125 mL (½ cup)

Leafy vegetables
Cooked:125 mL (½ cup)
Raw: 250 mL (1 cup)

Fresh, frozen or canned fruits
1 fruit or 125 mL (½ cup)

100% Juice
125 mL (½ cup)

Bread
1 slice (35 g)

Bagel
½ bagel (45 g)

Flat breads
½ pita or ½ tortilla (35 g)

Cooked rice, bulgur or quinoa
125 mL (½ cup)

Cereal
Cold: 30 g
Hot: 175 mL (¾ cup)

Cooked pasta or couscous
125 mL (½ cup)

Milk or powdered milk (reconstituted)
250 mL (1 cup)

Canned milk (evaporated)
125 mL (½ cup)

Fortified soy beverage
250 mL (1 cup)

Yogurt
175 g (¾ cup)

Kefir
175 g (¾ cup)

Cheese
50 g (1 ½ oz.)

Cooked fish, shellfish, poultry, lean meat
75 g (2 ½ oz.)/125 mL (½ cup)

Cooked legumes
175 mL (¾ cup)

Tofu
150 g or 175 mL (¾ cup)

Eggs
2 eggs

Peanut or nut butters
30 mL (2 Tbsp)

Shelled nuts and seeds
60 mL (¼ cup)

Oils and Fats
• Include a small amount – 30 to 45 mL (2 to 3 Tbsp) – of unsaturated fat each day. This includes oil used for cooking, salad dressings, margarine and mayonnaise.
• Use vegetable oils such as canola, olive and soybean.
• Choose soft margarines that are low in saturated and trans fats.
• Limit butter, hard margarine, lard and shortening.

Make each Food Guide Serving count...
wherever you are – at home, at school, at work or when eating out!

▶ **Eat at least one dark green and one orange vegetable each day.**
- Go for dark green vegetables such as broccoli, romaine lettuce and spinach.
- Go for orange vegetables such as carrots, sweet potatoes and winter squash.

▶ **Choose vegetables and fruit prepared with little or no added fat, sugar or salt.**
- Enjoy vegetables steamed, baked or stir-fried instead of deep-fried.

▶ **Have vegetables and fruit more often than juice.**

▶ **Make at least half of your grain products whole grain each day.**
- Eat a variety of whole grains such as barley, brown rice, oats, quinoa and wild rice.
- Enjoy whole grain breads, oatmeal or whole wheat pasta.

▶ **Choose grain products that are lower in fat, sugar or salt.**
- Compare the Nutrition Facts table on labels to make wise choices.
- Enjoy the true taste of grain products. When adding sauces or spreads, use small amounts.

▶ **Drink skim, 1%, or 2% milk each day.**
- Have 500 mL (2 cups) of milk every day for adequate vitamin D.
- Drink fortified soy beverages if you do not drink milk.

▶ **Select lower fat milk alternatives.**
- Compare the Nutrition Facts table on yogurts or cheeses to make wise choices.

▶ **Have meat alternatives such as beans, lentils and tofu often.**

▶ **Eat at least two Food Guide Servings of fish each week.***
- Choose fish such as char, herring, mackerel, salmon, sardines and trout.

▶ **Select lean meat and alternatives prepared with little or no added fat or salt.**
- Trim the visible fat from meats. Remove the skin on poultry.
- Use cooking methods such as roasting, baking or poaching that require little or no added fat.
- If you eat luncheon meats, sausages or prepackaged meats, choose those lower in salt (sodium) and fat.

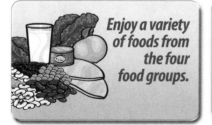

Enjoy a variety of foods from the four food groups.

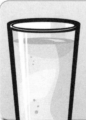

Satisfy your thirst with water!

Drink water regularly. It's a calorie-free way to quench your thirst. Drink more water in hot weather or when you are very active.

* Health Canada provides advice for limiting exposure to mercury from certain types of fish. Refer to www.healthcanada.gc.ca for the latest information.

Appendix II: Resources

Recommended Books

The Good Food Book for Families, by Brenda Bradshaw
and Cheryl Mutch
Published by Random House Canada

Your Child's Best Shot: A Parent's Guide to Vaccination,
by Ronald Gold, MD, MPH
Published by the Canadian Paediatric Society:
www.cps.ca/english/publications/Bookstore

Resource Books from the American Academy of Pediatrics:
Caring for Your Baby and Young Child
Your Baby's First Year

Websites

American Academy of Allergy, Asthma and Immunology
www.aaaai.org

American Academy of Pediatrics
www.aap.org

American Dietetic Association
www.eatright.org

Anemia Institute
www.anemiainstitute.org

Best Start Resource Center
www.beststart.org

British Columbia Medical Association
www.bcma.org/special-projects

Canadian Dental Association
www.cda-adc.ca

Canadian Food Inspection Agency
www.inspection.gc.ca

Canadian Paediatric Society
www.cps.ca

Canada's Physical Activity Guide
www.phac-aspc.gc.ca/pau-uap/paguide

Centers for Disease Control and Prevention
www.cdc.gov

Childhood Obesity Foundation
www.childhoodobesityfoundation.ca

Dial-A-Dietician
www.dialadietician.org

Dieticians of Canada
www.dieticians.ca

Environment Canada
Mercury and the Environment: Fish Consumption
http://www.ec.gc.ca/MERCURY/EN/fc.cfm

Eating Well with Canada's Food Guide
www.hc-sc.gc.ca/fn-an/food-guide-aliment/index_e.html

Eating Well with Canada's Food Guide: First Nations, Inuit and Métis
www.hc-sc.gc.ca/fn-an/pubs/fnim-pnim/index-eng.php

Gluten Intolerance/Coeliac Disease Support
www.coeliac.org.uk

HealthLink BC
www.healthlinkbc.ca

Health Canada
www.hc-sc.gc.ca

La Leche League
www.llli.org

Leslie Beck, RD
www.lesliebeck.com

National Center for Health Statistics: Centers for Disease Control
and Prevention Growth Charts
www.cdc.gov/growthcharts/

Author website
www.goodfoodbooksforkids.com

The National Institute of Health / National Institute of Digestive
Diseases (U.S.)
For information on lactose intolerance.
**http://digestive.niddk.nih.gov/ddiseases/pubs/
lactoseintolerance/index.htm**

Ontario Ministry of Health and Long-term Care
Sport Fish Contaminant Monitoring Program
**http://www.health.gov.on.ca/english/public/pub/foodsafe/
sportfish.html**

The Vitamin D Society
www.vitamindsociety.org

St. John Ambulance
http://www.sja.ca

Appendix III:
Growth Charts

The following are growth charts from the U.S. Centers for Disease Control. The charts are based on large population studies and are independent of race and ethnicity. They also include both breastfed and formula-fed infants. To plot your baby's progress, choose either the male or female chart and find the age in months on the horizontal axis and trace up to the height or weight on the vertical axis. The point plotted corresponds to a "growth percentile." For example, a male baby found to be in the 75 percent range for height is taller than 75 percent of all male babies his age and shorter than 25 percent of all male babies his age. Growth generally follows along a percentile curve throughout infancy. Concerns arise when growth is below or above expected percentiles or when growth deviates from predicted patterns.

Birth to 36 months: Boys
Length-for-age and Weight-for-age percentiles

NAME _____

RECORD # _____

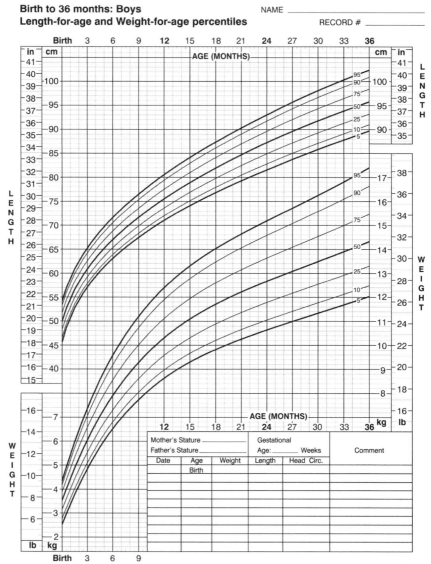

Published May 30, 2000 (modified 4/20/01).
SOURCE: Developed by the National Center for Health Statistics in collaboration with
the National Center for Chronic Disease Prevention and Health Promotion (2000).
http://www.cdc.gov/growthcharts

SAFER · HEALTHIER · PEOPLE™

Birth to 36 months: Girls
Length-for-age and Weight-for-age percentiles

NAME _____

RECORD # _____

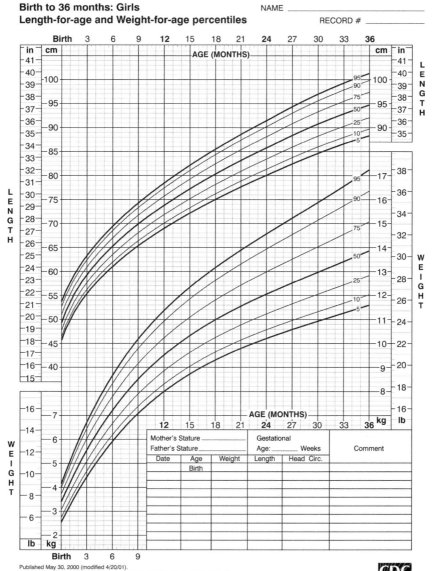

Published May 30, 2000 (modified 4/20/01).
SOURCE: Developed by the National Center for Health Statistics in collaboration with
the National Center for Chronic Disease Prevention and Health Promotion (2000).
http://www.cdc.gov/growthcharts

SAFER · HEALTHIER · PEOPLE™

Appendix IV:
References

1. Canadian Paediatric Society, Dietitians of Canada and Health Canada. Nutrition for Healthy Term Infants. Ottawa: Minister of Public Works and Government Services; 2005. Revised 2006.

2. Health Canada. Exclusive Breastfeeding Duration: 2004. Health Canada Recommendations, 2004.

3. American Academy of Pediatrics Work Group on Breastfeeding Policy Statement. Breastfeeding and the use of human milk (RE9729). *Pediatrics.* 1997;100:1035–1039.

4. Beaudry M et al. Relationship between infant feeding and infections during the first six months of life. *J. Pediatr.* 1995;126:191–197.

5. Ford RPK, Taylor BJ, Mitchell EA. Breastfeeding and the risk of sudden infant death syndrome. *Int J Epidemiol.* 1993;22:885–890.

6. Horwood LJ and Ferguson DM. Breastfeeding and later cognitive development and academic outcomes. *Pediatrics.* 1998;101:9.

7. Temboury et al. Influence of breastfeeding on the infant's intellectual development. *J. Pediatr Gastroenter Nutr.* 1994;18:32–36.

8. Chandra RK. Five year follow-up of high risk infants with family history of allergy who were exclusively breast-fed or fed partial whey hydrosylate, soy, and conventional cow's milk formulas. *J Pediatr Gastroenterol Nutr.* 1997;24:380–388.

9. Saarinen UM, Kajosaari M. Breastfeeding as prophylaxis against atopic disease: prospective follow-up study until 17 years old. *Lancet.* 1995;346:1065–1069.

10. Greene-Finestone L, Feldman W, Heick H, et al. Prevalence and risk factors of iron depletion and iron deficiency anaemia among infants in Ottawa-Carlton. *Can Diet Assoc J.* 1991;52:20–23.

11. Pizarro F, Yip R, Dallman PR, et al. Iron status with different infant feeding regimens: relevance to screening and prevention of iron deficiency. *J Pediatr.* 1991;118:687–692.

12. Cumming RG, Klineberg RJ. Breastfeeding and other reproductive factors and the risk of hip fractures in elderly women. *Int J Epidemiol.* 1993;22:684–691.

13. Melton LJ et al. Influence of breastfeeding and other reproductive factors on bone mass later in life. *Osteopros Int.* 1993;3:76–83.

14. Newcomb PA et al. Lactation and reduced risk of premenopausal breast cancer. *N Engl J Med.* 1994;330:81–87.

15. Rosenblatt KA, Thomas DB. WHO collaborative study of neoplasia and steroid contraceptives. *Int J Epidemiol.* 1993;22:192–197.

16. Dewey et al. Maternal weight-loss patterns during prolonged lactation. *Am J Clin Nutr.* 1993;58:162–166.

17. Canadian Paediatric Society, Indian and Inuit Health Committee. Vitamin D supplementation for northern native communities. *Can Med Assoc J.* 1988;138:229–230.

18. Lawrence et al. Prevention of rickets and vitamin D deficiency. New guidelines for vitamin D intake. *Pediatrics.* 2003;111:908–910.

19. Health Canada. Vitamin D Supplementation for Breastfed Infants: 2004. Health Canada Recommendations, 2004.

20. Lawton ME. Alcohol in breastmilk. *Aust NewZeal J Obstet Gynaecol.* 1985;25:71–73.

21. Little RE et al. Maternal alcohol use during breast-feeding and infant mental and motor development at one year. *New Engl J Med.* 1989;7:425–430.

22. Menella JA, Gerrish CJ. Effects of exposure to alcohol in mother's milk on infant sleep. *Pediatrics.* 1998;101(5):2.

23. Canadian Institute of Child Health. National breastfeeding guidelines for health care providers. 2nd ed., Ottawa; 1996.

24. Smith MM, Lifshitz F. Excess fruit juice consumption as a contributing factor in nonorganic failure to thrive. *Pediatrics.* 1994;93:438–443.

25. Canadian Paediatric Society, Nutrition Committee. The use of fluoride in infants and children. *Paediatrics & Child Health.* 2002;7(8):569–572. Reference no. N02–01. Revision in progress February, 2009.

26. Lucassen et al. Effectiveness of treatments for infantile colic: systematic review. *BMJ.* 1998;316:1563–1569.

27. The American Academy of Pediatrics. *Guide to Your Child's Nutrition.* New York: Random House, 1999.

28. HealthlinkBC. Child Nutrition Series File #69b. Formula Feeding Your Baby; Safely Preparing and Storing Formula. 2006.

29. HealthlinkBC. Child Nutrition Series File #69c. Baby's First Foods. 2007.

30. Greer F et al. Effects of Early Nutritional Interventions on The Development of Atopic Disease in Infants and Children: The Role of Maternal Dietary Restriction, Breastfeeding, Timing of Introduction of Complementary Foods, and Hydrolyzed Formulas. *Pediatrics.* 2008;121:183–191.

31. Sicherer S, Burks W. Maternal and infant diets for prevention of allergic diseases: Understanding menu changes in 2008. *Journal of Allergy and Clinical Immunology.* 2008;122:29–33.

32. Canadian Paediatric Society. Fatal anaphylactic reactions to food in children. *Can Med Assoc J.* 1994;150:337–339.

33. Bloomfield SF et al. Too clean or not too clean: the hygiene hypothesis and home hygiene. *Clinical and Experimental Allergy.* 2006;31(4):402–425.

34. Dewey et al. Breastfed infants are leaner than formula fed infants at one year of age: The Darling Study. *Am J Clin Nutr.* 1993;57:140–145.

35. Canadian Paediatric Society and Health Canada. Report of the Joint Working Group. Nutrition Recommendations Update: Dietary Fat and Children. Ottawa. 1994.

36. Pickering et al. Modulation of the immune system by human milk and infant formula containing nucleotides. *Pediatrics.* 1998;101:242–249.

37. Schutze GE et al. The home environment and salmonellosis in children. *Pediatrics.* 1999;103:1.

38. Canadian Paediatric Society. Meeting the needs of infants and young children: an update. *Can Med Assoc J.* 1991;144:1451–1454.

39. Government of Canada. Questions and answers for action on Bisphenol A under the chemicals management plan. October 2008.

40. HealthLinkBC. Nutrition Series File #68m. Healthy Eating: Choose Fish Low in Mercury. 2007.

41. Feldman W, Randel P. Screening children for lead exposure in Canada. In: Canadian Task Force on the Periodic Health Examination. Canadian Guide to Clinical Preventative Health Care. Ottawa: Health Canada; 1994;268–288.

42. Canadian Paediatric Society. Effective discipline for children. *Paediatrics & Child Health.* 1997;2(1):29–33.

43. Hodge et al. Consumption of oily fish and childhood asthma risk. *MJA.* 1996;164:137–140.

44. Stevens et al. Omega-3 fatty acids and boys with behaviour, learning and health problems. *Physiology and Behaviour.* 1996;59:915–920.

45. American Academy of Pediatrics Provisional Committee on Quality Improvement, Subcommittee on Acute Gastroenteritis. Practice parameter: the management of acute gastroenteritis in young children. *Pediatrics.* 1996;97:424–435.

46. Canadian Paediatric Society, Nutrition Committee. Oral rehydration therapy and early refeeding in the management of gastroenteritis. *Can J Paediatr.* 1994b;1:160–164.

47. Yagev Y, Koren G. Eating fish during pregnancy, risk of exposure to toxic levels of methylmercury. *Canadian Family Physician.* 2002;48:1619–1621.

48. Health Canada. Information Update. Health Canada advises specific groups to limit their consumption of canned albacore tuna. February 2007.

49. Health Canada. Information Update. Health Canada's revised assessment of mercury in fish enhances protection while reflecting advice in Canada's Food Guide. March 2007.

50. Health Canada. Food and Nutrition. Mercury in Fish. February 2008.

51. Hites et al. Global assessment of organic contaminants in farmed salmon. *Science.* 2004;303:226–229.

52. Craig-Schmidt MC. Isomeric fatty acids: evaluating status and implications for maternal and child health. *Lipids.* 2001;36:997–1006.

53. Health Canada. Drugs and Health Products. Questions and Answers—Hormonal Growth Promoters. 2005.

Recipe Index

General Index

ADHD (attention deficit hyper-
    activity disorder), 96
Alcohol, 13
Allergies. *See also* Food intolerances
    and breastfeeding, 6
    common food, 29
    to cow's milk, 6, 15, 32
    diagnosis of food, 30
    to eggs, 32, 111
    family history of food, 6, 30–31
    and hygiene theory, 30
    and introduction of solid food,
        24–28, 31
    management of food, 31–34
    to peanuts, 31, 62
    prevalence of food, 28
    severe food, 31
    to soy, 14–15, 29, 33, 104
    to wheat, 27, 33, 100, 106
Anaphylaxis, 31, 33
Anemia. *See* Iron-deficiency anemia
Antioxidants, 39, 41
Appetite, 122
    poor or decreased, 84, 109, 151

of toddlers, 141, 155, 156
and zinc in diet, 100
Apple juice, unpasteurized, 76
Asthma, 6, 94
Attention deficit hyperactivity
    disorder (ADHD), 96

Baby food. *See* Solid food
Beans, 97
Beta-carotene, 41
Bisphenol A, 10–11
    in baby bottles, 10–11
Blueberries, disease-fighting
    properties of, 57
Blood in stool, 73, 76, 151
Bone development, 9, 39, 65, 123
Bottle
    nipples, 16
    self-feeding with, 109
    sterilization of, 16
    switching to cup from, 109, 162
    used as pacifier, 109
Bowel diseases, reducing risk of, 6

ACKNOWLEDGMENTS

We would like to thank a number of people whose help and support contributed greatly to this book: Dr. Cheryl Mutch, Anne Lindsay, Karen Fryer, Val Bradshaw, Elaine Donaldson, Dr. Richard Goldbloom and Random House Canada. As well, thanks to Corrinne Eisler at the Vancouver Coastal Health Authority for her continued guidance. A special thanks goes to Linda Kirste at Dial-A-Dietitian for patiently taking the time to answer our questions. To our husbands, Craig Bramley and Jeff Petter, we are grateful for your love and support.

BRENDA BRADSHAW is an elementary school teacher living in Vancouver. She is co-author of *The Good Food Book for Families*, an avid cook, and the mother of two.

DR. LAUREN DONALDSON BRAMLEY is a registered doctor in Australia, Canada, China and Hong Kong. Dr. Bramley now practices in Hong Kong where she lives with her husband and three children.